Central Auditory Processing Disorder

Strategies for Use with Children and Adolescents

Dorothy A. Kelly,
D.A., CCC-SLP

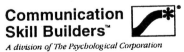

Communication Skill Builders™

A division of The Psychological Corporation

555 Academic Court
San Antonio, Texas 78204
800-228-0752

Reproducing Pages from This Book

As described below, some of the pages in this book may be reproduced for instructional or administrative use (not for resale). To protect your book, make a photocopy of each reproducible page. Then use that copy as a master for photocopying.

About the Author

Dorothy A. Kelly is an assistant professor in the Department of Speech Communication, St. Joseph's College, Patchogue, New York. A speech-language pathologist and teacher of hearing-impaired children and adults, she is an editorial consultant and writer for *ADVANCE for Speech-Language Pathologists and Audiologists;* is consultant practitioner to Suffolk County's Early Intervention Services Program; and maintains a small private practice for diagnosis, therapy, and consultations in South Setauket, New York. Previous experiences include supervision of the Speech-Language Department at Just Kids Early Learning Center, Middle Island, New York; teacher of the hearing impaired at Mill Neck Manor School for the Deaf, Mill Neck, New York; and consultant to The Institute for Behavioral Health, Commack, New York.

Dorothy A. Kelly received the doctor of arts degree in Communicative Disorders from Adelphi University; the master of arts degree in Speech-Language Pathology and Audiology from Hofstra University; and the bachelor of science degree in Deaf Education/Elementary/Nursery Education from State University College of New York at Buffalo; with additional credits from C. W. Post College and Pace University.

Dr. Kelly holds permanent New York State certification in Speech and Hearing Handicapped, Classes for the Deaf, and Elementary/Nursery Education; and she is licensed in New York State as a Speech-Language Pathologist. She holds the American Speech-Language-Hearing Association's Certificate of Clinical Competence.

This book is dedicated to my two children,
Laura and Kevin Cassar, who endured endless
computer breakdowns, revisions, and
distractions for months without complaint.
They are my support, my joy, and my inspiration.
Children are what it's all about.

Acknowledgments

If it were not for the interest and support I received from Kenneth Kaufman, Ph.D., director of the Institute for Behavioral Health, this book probably would not have been written—or at the very least, would not be in its present form. At a time when it seemed that there was confusion about central auditory processing disorders in children experiencing academic, social, and language difficulties, Dr. Kaufman was eager to identify, to learn, and to share information. I have benefitted tremendously from our association.

I would also like to thank all the parents and children with whom I have worked—especially those families who had concerns about central auditory processing disorders.

Thanks also to all the classroom teachers with open hearts and minds. They have added to the process immeasurably.

Contents

PART ONE
The Child with Central Auditory
Processing Disorder

Chapter 1. Overview

PART TWO
Diagnosis

Chapter 2. Foundations for Diagnosis

PART FOUR
Intervention and Remediation

PART FIVE
Transition and Carryover

APPENDIX, GLOSSARY, REFERENCES

Preface

In my twenty-plus years of experience as a speech-language pathologist and teacher of the hearing impaired, I have had the good fortune to work in a number of educational and clinical settings, including nursery, elementary, and high schools, nursing homes, hospitals, health departments, group homes, schools for the deaf, special education facilities, and so-called "normal" classrooms. This range of experience has afforded me opportunity to observe individuals with central auditory processing disorders in various forms. I have grown to realize how highly individualized and widespread the phenomena can be.

Twenty years ago, the term *central auditory processing* was a mysterious and somewhat controversial term that tended to send shivers up the spines of clinicians. Because of the enigma surrounding the disorder and the lack of clear-cut definitions and criteria, many children were mislabeled or not labeled at all. Often the child with central auditory processing disorder (CAPD) was thought to be learning disabled, hearing impaired, or a behavior problem.

We have made considerable gains; but the reality in many educational settings is that we still are not quite sure how to identify, assess, and remediate the child with CAPD. In some children we still are not certain how central auditory processing disorders fit into the larger issues of attention deficit disorder, learning disabilities, dyslexia, and hearing impairment.

Inspired by those children who "fall through the cracks," I will address some of these issues and raise a few others. Practical, pragmatic procedures for identification and intervention are provided in an effort to facilitate the tasks ahead for parent, teacher, speech-language pathologist, and student.

Introduction

In this book, no attempt has been made to provide an in-depth analysis of various theories of information processing or hearing. Such discussion, although critical, would be better left to more theoretical efforts. Rather, the major focus here is to provide essential information regarding the behavioral effects of central auditory processing deficiencies on language and language-dependent performance in both academic and social settings. This book further provides specific suggestions and therapy materials with which to improve functioning. Throughout the book, reproducible forms and handouts are made available. It is hoped that in this way the speech-language pathologist will be able to "fine tune" theoretical skills into practical and immediate applications.

The issue of disorder versus delay in language functioning has been debated in the literature for quite some time. In this book, we will examine the question of delay (suggesting a largely quantitative difference in functioning) versus disorder (suggesting a qualitative or "disordered" difference in functioning) in central auditory processing assessment. Differences among children may exist in the acquisition and status of skills. For example, the environmentally deprived child who may not have been exposed to varied and consistent opportunities to build auditory memory or discrimination skills may appear different from the child who perhaps has had such opportunities but was unable to make use of them effectively. These distinctions may be helpful in terms of identification as well as intervention strategies. Future research may explore such questions and subsequently provide clearer theoretical philosophies.

This book is divided into five major sections:

Part One: The Child with Central Auditory Processing Disorder

Part Two: Diagnosis

Part Three: Practical Suggestions for Parents, Teachers, and Students

Part Four: Intervention and Remediation

Part Five: Transition and Carryover

Practical information is presented regarding identification, management, and remediation of the child with central auditory processing disorder. In viewing the "total" child, suggestions are offered to the student, teacher, and parent. It is hoped that the information provided will decrease the likelihood of these children "falling through the cracks" in a highly complex and overburdened educational system.

Before You Begin

Before you begin, you may want to compile "CAP PACS" for the student, parent, teacher, and yourself, using all appropriate reproducible materials in this book. Select materials from Part Three (Practical Suggestions for Parents, Teachers, and Students) and from other areas as indicated. (All reproducible materials are listed and identified in the Contents, pages vii-xii.) Place these materials in a folder, and use them for ongoing monitoring, reminders, charts, documentation, and other purposes.

PART ONE

The Child with Central Auditory Processing Disorder

Part One provides general information regarding central auditory processing disorder, such as definitions, etiological factors, psychological factors, and correlates to language functioning. It is designed to identify the child with CAPD from several perspectives.

1
Overview

What Are Central Auditory Processing Disorders?

In 1992, the American Speech-Language-Hearing Association's Ad Hoc Committee on Central Auditory Processing issued this definition:*

> Central auditory processing disorders are deficits in the information processing of audible signals not attributed to impaired peripheral hearing sensitivity or intellectual impairment. This information processing involves perceptual, cognitive, and linguistic functions that, with appropriate interaction, result in effective receptive communication of auditorily presented stimuli. Specifically, CAPD refers to limitations in the ongoing transmission, analysis, organization, transformation, elaboration, storage, retrieval, and use of information contained in audible signals. CAPD may involve the listener's active and passive (e.g., conscious and unconscious, mediated and unmediated, controlled and automatic) ability to do the following:
>
> > attend, discriminate, and identify acoustic signals;
> >
> > transform and continuously transmit information through both the peripheral and central nervous systems;
> >
> > filter, sort, and combine information at appropriate perceptual and conceptual levels;
> >
> > store and retrieve information efficiently; restore, organize, and use retrieved information;
> >
> > segment and decode acoustic stimuli using phonological, semantic, syntactic, and pragmatic knowledge; and
> >
> > attach meaning to a stream of acoustic signals through the use of linguistic and nonlinguistic contexts.

Central auditory processing has been described by Lasky and Katz (1983, 4) as the manipulation and utilization of sound signals by the central nervous system. Boone (1987, 100-101) identifies central auditory processing dysfunction as

---

*Reprinted by permission of the American Speech-Language-Hearing Association

"difficulty in processing and understanding both nonverbal and verbal auditory stimuli . . . believed to be the result of auditory stimuli reaching the brain with inadequate processing of the perceived stimuli."

Bernice Heasley (1974, 19-32), one of the earlier authors on the topic of central auditory processing, offered perhaps the most comprehensive taxonomy. She identified fourteen processing skills:

1. Awareness of sound

2. Auditory attention

3. Auditory attention span

4. Localization of sound

5. Discrimination for sound

6. Auditory memory

7. Auditory memory span

8. Auditory sequencing ability

9. Auditory projection

10. Auditory separation

11. Auditory blending

12. Auditory closure

13. Subvocalization

14. Reauditorization

Simply stated, central auditory processing involves what we do with what we hear. Competency in processing requires an intact auditory signal, an intact ear, an intact auditory nerve, and a brain that is able to receive the information and act upon it meaningfully. It is a phenomenon involving a range of behaviors from awareness of the presence of sound to higher-order analysis of linguistic information. Deficits in central auditory processing may range from mild to severe and may involve a single behavior or skill area or a combination of skill areas. These skills are several in number and may be known by more than one term. They include, but are not limited to, auditory memory, auditory discrimination, and auditory figure-ground. Individuals with central auditory processing disorders are a widely defined, highly heterogeneous group.

Normal processing development appears contingent upon three main factors:

1. Intact auditory peripheral and nervous systems

2. Variety of intact and repeated auditory experiences

3. Fundamental cognitive potentials

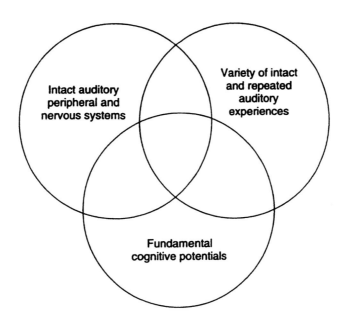

Figure 1. Components for Normal Central Auditory Processing Development

Skill Areas

For the purposes of this book, five main skill areas are identified which are believed to impact most significantly upon language, social, and academic performances. These skill areas are:

- *Auditory Memory*—The ability to recall auditory sequences in various forms such as words, numbers, and sentences. This skill area should not be thought of as only the ability to recall information immediately. Children may be able to recall sequences of numbers but not words, or perhaps can recall sentences but not nonrelated word sequences. Others may be able to recall all (or some) of the members of a sequence, but not in order. Others may not be able to retain the information over time. Furthermore, a good auditory memory does not necessarily mean that a child will be able to interpret and act upon a direction.

- *Auditory Discrimination*—The ability to note phonemic differences in words. This skill may involve identification of specific phonemes as well as recognition of sameness or difference. This skill area has apparent implications for spelling, reading, and following directions. A child may be able to identify phonemic differences within words but be unable to identify differences on a single phoneme basis. Some contrasts appear easier to identify than others. For example, discrimination between stop consonants such as /t/ versus /p/ is more challenging than discrimination between /l/ versus /s/. In this case, voicing and timing cues appear to make the task easier. This skill area, which may be present at birth, also appears related to the area of auditory perception (see pages 150-151).

- *Auditory Figure-Ground*—The ability to screen out ambient noise distractions or to focus upon a primary signal in the presence of secondary signals. The absence of this skill is troublesome in the classroom where background noises are common. Problems are compounded for the child who also has difficulties with auditory memory and interpretation of directions under ideal circumstances. This child often prefers one-to-one settings and is uncomfortable in group contexts. Auditory figure-ground is also known as auditory separation and auditory selective attention. Intensity, frequency, and meaningfulness of the distraction appear to impact upon performance.

- *Auditory Cohesion*—The ability to organize, interpret, and process on a higher-order level, wherein information may not be easily discernible on the surface. This skill often involves the processing of more sophisticated linguistic structures and appears to have some cognitive correlates. This skill may be in part dependent upon the development of lower-order processing skills such as auditory memory and discrimination. Auditory cohesion, as defined here, seems to be a skill which is somewhat developmental in nature in children, appearing to varying degrees of performance level at varying points in development.

- *Auditory Attention*—The ability to maintain purposeful auditory focus over an extended period of time. This is a skill which appears to be developmental to some degree and may involve several considerations. Issues of interest and volitionality arise; that is, even when the child is not interested in the auditory stimuli, is the child "able" to maintain attention as needed to complete the task? Conversely, when a child has "tuned out" or has become distracted, is it because of choice (the child became bored or uninterested) or because of an inability to maintain focus? Clearly, this issue becomes very critical when dealing with children who have attention deficit disorder as well as other children in which the concern for neurological status arises. Auditory attention, for the purposes of this book, is treated as a fifth auditory skill because of its clear impact upon classroom and social performance. However, auditory attention may not be a separate skill area as much as it is a phenomenon related to a number of other factors such as maturity, personality, learning style, and neurological status.

Auditory perception is another term appearing in central auditory processing literature and described in various manners. It will be discussed in greater detail at a later point (see pages 150-151).

References will be made to its possible relationship to auditory discrimination, among other areas of central auditory processing.

Figure 2 describes the hierarchical relationships among the five skill areas, suggesting a type of "building blocks" phenomenon.

Development of processing skills, as depicted in figure 3, may be viewed as an intricate process involving many dynamics.

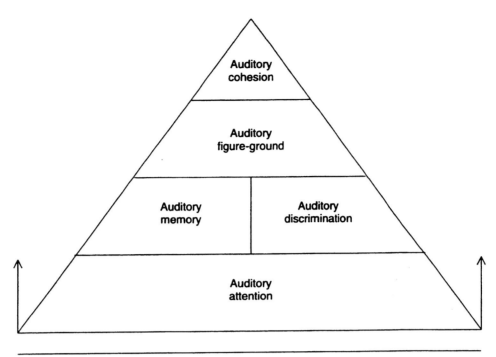

Figure 2. Suggested Hierarchy of Auditory Processing Skill Areas

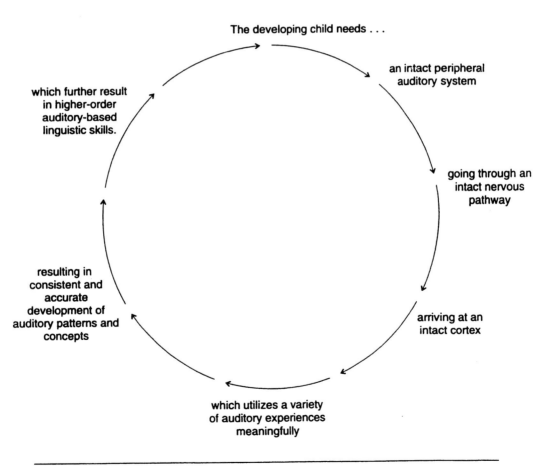

Figure 3. Normal Central Auditory Processing Development

Developmental Expectations

Questions regarding developmental expectations arise whenever therapy programs are designed. These issues are often debatable, but even more so in the area of central auditory processing dysfunction. Research sometimes raises more questions than it answers, particularly when it tries to define such terms as *perception* and *processing*. In reality, we do not know with certainty which skills are present at birth (and in what forms) and which skills develop later. The fruition of "developmental" skills is highly dependent upon factors such as status of hearing and health, as well as the consistency and quality of auditory experiences. Interestingly, we know that many children who are later diagnosed as having central auditory processing impairment respond appropriately to auditory stimuli for the first year or so of life, while others appear to evidence difficulties as newborns. While our research knowledge is growing, in some ways we really know less than what we *don't* know in this yet murky area.

"Normalcy" involves a range of performance that varies to some extent from one person to another. In any classroom, individual students will display varying levels of proficiency in auditory perceptual tasks involving discrimination, memory, cohesion, and other skills. When individual profiles of students are compared, differences again become apparent. Within the "typical" or "normal" population, there are no exact or clearly defined expectations. The typical person comes to "compensate" or balance weaker skills with stronger ones, achieving a kind of processing homeostasis or righting mechanism.

Etiological Factors

In individuals with central auditory processing dysfunction, the difficulty is not specific to the peripheral ear system. Hearing sensitivity, as tested by conventional pure-tone audiometry, is usually considered normal. Neurological findings tend to be unremarkable (Willeford 1985, 242). Some etiological factors, however, have been associated with central auditory processing dysfunction. These may be collectively cited as: brain tumor or abscess, vascular changes in the brain, brain damage resulting from trauma, kernicterus (bile deposits in the central nervous system), eighth cranial nerve damage, chronic incidence of otitis media (minimal auditory deficiency syndrome), lead poisoning, and malfunctioning of the corpus callosum (Newby 1972, 57; Pinheiro and Musiek 1985, 213, 214, 259; Martin 1986, 322-324; Wyngaarden 1987, 168).

Central auditory processing disorders may appear as primary or secondary diagnoses. For example, in neurologically related syndromes such as learning disability and attention deficit disorder, processing disorders may appear as a secondary condition. Some children with specific language-impairment (SLI) may display underlying deficits in central auditory processing (Tallal and Stark 1981). Willeford (1985, 242) states that auditory communication disorder is the common characteristic throughout a highly heterogeneous CAPD population.

In this book we will not attempt to clarify issues concerning the relationship between central auditory processing and various types of language disorders. Broad summaries of current views will be noted at a later point (see pages 13-14).

More simply, this book views auditory perceptual skills as tools or foundation skills that facilitate the acquisition of language and language-dependent behaviors such as reading and spelling. By being provided with these foundation skills, the child will be better able to acquire language naturally. The emphasis of therapy is to provide skills that can be applied practically to tasks, so that the child eventually learns to cope or function independently.

Comparison to Hearing Impairment

A question arises regarding individuals who are born with impaired hearing. Obviously, the degree and type of loss is critical, with severe or profound sensorineural losses being most significant. However, individuals born with impaired hearing may well suffer on both acuity (ear-based) and perceptual levels. Because the ear has not effectively sent an intact signal through the auditory nervous system, the opportunity for perceptual development has been thwarted. Thus, skills such as auditory memory and auditory figure-ground, which become more sophisticated over time with uncorrupted experiences, may not develop properly even in individuals with mild-to-moderate hearing impairment. Because the ear failed to work properly, the brain did not receive repeated, consistent, and reliable signals which would have facilitated perceptual growth. Children with less significant losses may display subtle perceptual deficits, particularly in the areas of auditory memory, discrimination, figure-ground, and cohesion.

Assessment becomes an important issue when peripheral hearing loss complicates the central processing profile. Many of the tests used to identify central auditory processing deficits cannot be used when a hearing loss has been identified. The specific impact of hearing loss (as opposed to perceptual deficit) upon test results is not yet clear and needs to be investigated further. Overlap may be possible on some assessment measures.

Psychological Factors

Children with CAPD must be viewed first as children, and then as children who have processing limitations. These children have the same emotional concerns as so-called "normal" children. Because children with CAPD have experienced "failure" on many levels at home as well as in school, often their self-esteem is minimal. Well-intentioned parents and teachers may try to address this deficit by telling the child that there isn't a problem and by denying the symptoms (for example, failure to maintain auditory focus or failure to follow directions). Sometimes the symptoms are assumed to be due to other factors ("He can pay attention when he wants to" or "She hears when she wants to"). Such mixed signals, however well meant, often confuse children with CAPD. It probably is best to identify difficulties in a direct yet empathetic manner, while providing strategies and plans for success.

Expectations placed on "normal" children by home and school are typically quite demanding. When children with CAPD try to measure up to such standards, often the experience is frustrating and emotionally debilitating, especially when the children don't really understand why they are "different" from their peers. Knowledge and understanding of the symptoms are critical to these children.

Over time, confusion and frustration often translate into "turning off and tuning out."

Children with low self-esteem often see academic challenges and social interaction as painful. These settings provide constant evidence that they are different and unsuccessful. The first hurdle to be crossed is to address attitude and self-image issues. Merely telling such children to do something in a certain way is not enough, whether in therapy or in the classroom. The children must be told *why* they are doing it in that particular manner and what positive results may be expected. The possible endpoints in therapy must be explained. Children also need to be told what their responsibilities are in therapy and what factors for change are within their control. It must be made clear to them that therapy is not a magic cure; it is only one factor toward reaching success. It won't work unless they actively and earnestly participate in their programs.

Children with CAPD make "choices" every day. They need to know that their difficulties in CAP are not an amorphous, overpowering phenomenon over which there is no control. Changes and strategies may be possible by dealing with problems head-on. These children must understand that they are not the CAP disorder; they are terrific, talented children who "choose" to accept the challenge that CAP presents.

This is not to say that the child or parent should be led to believe that a "miracle cure" is possible. We really don't know with certainty how many processing disorders mature. If they are neurophysiological in nature, it appears likely that the child won't simply "grow out of it." However, we do know that many children acquire coping strategies that allow them to succeed in a variety of settings.

Partnerships between parent and child, teacher and child, must be formed in which members contribute ideas and cooperate toward a common goal. The quality of the rapport between therapist and child is critical in this type of intervention. When the child sees the therapist as not only an authority figure but someone who respects the child's input and who is on the same team, progress is more assured. A child who feels empowered toward achieving an important goal will become more dedicated to its realization. Success breeds success; all gains must be acknowledged.

Theoretical Approaches

Professionals who approach central auditory processing disorders can be broadly divided into two groups: those who ascribe to language-based origins, and those who maintain that disorders are auditory-perceptual or signal-based in nature. Those clinicians who believe that CAPDs are generally higher-order and language-based describe symptoms in terms such as auditory closure, auditory analysis, and auditory memory. Deficits are viewed in terms of their linguistic dependency. Observations are made in relationship to linguistically dependent tasks such as reading, writing, and spelling. Speech-language pathologists generally support this theoretical perspective.

Audiologists often support the view that CAPDs are auditory-perceptually based and involve a breakdown somewhere in the auditory nervous system. Descriptions of symptoms may include auditory discrimination scores, dichotic listening skills, and signal-to-noise ratios. Assessment procedures often involve, but are not limited to, site of lesion testing.

Two approaches to intervention, rooted in recent developments in cognitive neuroscience, arise when auditory processing is correlated with language processing and directionality. "Bottom-up" processing is inductive in nature and suggests that a process begins with basic data and is elevated upward. The structure of language enables us to understand without having to decode individual sounds or words. Bottom-up, acoustic input processes enable the listener to respond to novel information or information that is less predictable.

The opposite view offers a "top-down" or deductive paradigm in which processing begins with higher-order conceptual information and then progresses to lower-order basic data. Top-down, knowledge-oriented processes enable the listener to respond to lower-order information that is more predictable and commonplace in terms of experience.

Information processing, which is multistage, interactive, and highly complex in nature, appears to involve both paradigms. Phonological, lexical, and syntactic cues provide top-down sources of information, while acoustic cues such as voice-onset time and segment duration provide bottom-up information. The listener, in this emerging view, uses both processes flexibly, depending upon need, relying on one more heavily than the other in particular listening tasks. For example, in noisy settings the listener may have to depend upon top-down processes more specifically because of the corrupted nature of the stimuli.

Diagnostic and intervention strategies vary according to the theoretical approach adopted. In this book, both perspectives are blended. Some central auditory processing tasks are complex in nature and result from both signal-based as well as higher-order linguistic problems, while others are more narrowly defined. This broad perspective is practical in terms of intervention for the many different types and displays of central auditory processing disorders.

Research in central auditory processing may be broadly divided between efforts directed at speech perception and those which address auditory perception. Psychoacoustic research (speech perception) often centers upon the sensitivity of the auditory system, while neurophysiologic research (auditory perception) generally deals with understanding how the properties of acoustic signals affect neurons in the auditory pathways (Sloan 1991, 6).

Correlates to Language Functioning

The relationship between central auditory processing and language performance has always been difficult to specify. How deficient processing skills impact on language performance is not simply quantified. For example, when a child performs poorly when compared to age-peers on a receptive comprehension test, is it due to true language impairment, central auditory processing dysfunction (that is, deficient foundation tools for language development), or both?

In some cases, children who display language difficulties in various forms also may display aspects of central auditory processing disorder. These children may actually have a dual diagnosis. It may serve well to examine such possibilities at the outset of therapy. If processing skills are found to be lacking, these needs then can be addressed early on and quite probably impact positively upon language acquisitions. Some children who are diagnosed as language impaired or learning disabled may have central auditory processing problems as either primary or secondary conditions (Eisenson 1966, 1972; Lubert 1981; Pinheiro 1977; Rosenthal 1977; Sloan 1980; Tallal 1980).

Paula Tallal, Ph.D., stated that CAPD is a major problem for children who eventually develop speaking and reading problems (Trace 1993a). CAPD children are at risk for phonological deficits as well. According to Tallal, data strongly suggests a neurophysiological aspect to processing disorders. She noted the possibility of a neurophysiological timing defect that negatively affects reading and spelling skills. The relationship between neurophysiology and central auditory processing has been investigated (Abbs and Sussman 1971; Delgutte 1980; Kiang 1980). When issues such as these are raised, the susceptibility of all language functions that are auditory processing-dependent becomes apparent.

Pragmatic development is an area of language functioning that is not frequently considered in terms of central auditory processing skills. A child who has difficulty with background noises, following conversations, or decoding similar sounding words may display pragmatic differences. These children's social experiences may be affected both quantitatively *(how much?)* and qualitatively *(in what way?)*. The child who has difficulty in conversations is not likely to engage in them freely and appropriately. This may be an intervention issue for children with CAPD who develop better processing skills in therapy but then need "fine-tuning" to learn how to apply these skills appropriately in social settings.

Reception problems are often related to expression problems. Thus, central auditory processing disorders may directly or indirectly affect other aspects of language functioning, including phonological development, receptive and expressive vocabulary, expressive language skills such as syntax and morphology, and receptive language comprehension. Because central auditory processing disorders may be primary or secondary conditions and may vary widely in terms of type and degree of severity, individual profiles will differ significantly. Successful intervention is dependent upon addressing all of these issues.

Age-Related Changes

Recent research has focused on the relationship between aging, hearing, and central auditory processes. James Jerger, Ph.D., CCC-A, and associates at Baylor College of Medicine in Houston have studied topographical brain mapping of auditorily evoked potentials. Brain mapping—the recoding of activity in various parts of the brain—is helpful in diagnosing and monitoring central auditory processing disorders in older patients. According to Jerger (Trace 1993b), aging often involves the progressive asymmetricalization of the brain. This breakdown results in lessened interhemispheric communication and can take the form of reduced ability to process auditory information. Jerger observed that many elderly patients, 65 to 70 years of age and older, have difficulty processing verbal information in their left ears and nonverbal information in their right ears. Overall, there appears to be a disportionate decline in communication and auditory functioning in the elderly, for which hearing aids are often of minimal benefit.

Interestingly, this apparent age-related degeneration of central auditory processing skills is in sharp contrast to the experiences of many children with CAPD. In the former case, skills which were intact at some earlier point have degenerated; while in the latter case, the issue is often more developmental or maturational (that is, possibly the skills were never intact).

Aging individuals evidence significant difficulties in signal-to-noise ratios even when hearing acuity is considered normal (Pinheiro and Musiek 1985, 259). Aging also appears to be associated with a decreased ability to respond to time cues, including the binaural cues used in localization. These difficulties are not accountable in terms of hearing loss alone, and appear to be perceptually based.

The American Speech-Language-Hearing Association addressed the concerns of central auditory processing and aging at its national convention in November, 1993. Raymond H. Hull, Ph.D., CCC-A, of the University of Northern Colorado, presented a poster session entitled Central Auditory Processing in Aging: Compounding Elements in Advancing Age. Hull identified and discussed factors of processing that appear to accompany aging and which can be further complicated in patients with hearing impairment. The elderly person with hearing impairment does not compensate for sensitivity losses as well as younger counterparts, due to poorer auditory processing skills (Trace 1993b).

Among other research findings, Hull noted a decline in the speed of auditory closure and synthesis with age. This "timing" difficulty relates both to perception of speech and cognitive processing. Hull found that the short-term memory deficits observed in some elderly patients may negatively impact on word analysis (Trace 1993b). Interestingly, Hull identified timing difficulties as being problematic in children with various learning disabilities as well.

In sum, our current understanding of age-related perceptual changes reflects a recognition of the interplay of cognitive-linguistic, central auditory, and peripheral auditory processes. These processes are dynamic and interdependent. Possible drug-related effects upon processing also should be noted; the aged population is one in which the use of prescription drugs is widespread.

Other questions arise with regard to age and readiness or receptivity to therapy. Is there a critical period in which a child can respond best to intervention? Is there a time that is too late? At various points in the research literature, critical learning periods have been identified for specific syndromes and disorders. Some of these time frames have held true, and some have been held up to further scrutiny.

While we do not have an abundance of research to document age prognosticators for central auditory processing disordered conditions, we can assume generally that younger students have more positive therapy outlooks. The central nervous system is viable by nature, capable of accommodation, and receptive to intervention (Musiek, Lenz, and Gollegly 1991). Maximum gains in therapy have been correlated with timeliness and early intervention. These findings, however, do not imply that the older individual should not engage in therapy or that progress is not possible. It simply indicates that certain candidacy factors should be evaluated when designing a course for intervention.

Research has provided us with other age predictors and parameters. Neuman and Hochberg (1983) found differences in syllable identification as a function of age. Additionally, they discovered that the ability to identify speech in reverberant environments improved with age up until age 13, when it achieved adult levels of performance. Northern and Lemme (1988, 434) suggested that many central auditory processing skills "grow" in early childhood and stabilize in the seventh or eighth year. Such developmental expectations should be incorporated into elementary school curricula and acknowledged in terms of classroom dynamics.

Sex Differences

The research has provided minimal information regarding possible sex differences in children with CAPDs. However, based on anecdotal reports from clinicians, case histories, case-load ratios, and other informal sources of information, it appears possible that boys are more at risk for CAPD than girls. Additionally, considering the fact that the corpus callosum or connecting bridge between the cortical hemispheres differs in size and shape in males and females, differences in processing are quite possible. Future research may seek to further specify such possible sex differences. Such information also may provide insights into possible sex-related processing differences in "normal" individuals.

Profiles in Childhood—Case Studies in CAPD

The following seven case studies typify diagnostic profiles of individuals with central auditory processing disorder. The first one is that of an adult male. This profile provides possible perspective in terms of adult behaviors and characteristics. The remaining six profiles are of children—five boys and one girl—ages three through 13 years. Parts of each diagnostic profile are italicized as a means of identifying possible "red flags" or areas of concern to the speech-language pathologist.

John B

John B was a bright, personable 27-year-old man who was currently being evaluated for attention deficit disorder by a behavioral psychologist. He was referred for central auditory processing evaluation by the psychologist based upon anecdotal reports concerning *difficulty with verbal directions, impulsivity,* and *figure-ground problems.* Mr. B reported that he dropped out of high school when he was 16 years old due to *reading difficulties* (dyslexia) and what he felt was an *inability to focus.* He indicated that he did not receive any special education services other than speech therapy for articulation errors in elementary school. According to Mr. B, all testing completed during his school years indicated *above-average intelligence,* and he recalled that his teachers were frustrated by his *apparent lack of effort.* He also recalled that he was taught reading via a sight = vocabulary approach and is *unable to decode words,* according to Mr. B, due to this "poor phonics background." Mr. B reported that he later received his G.E.D. diploma and had subsequently attempted to complete several correspondence courses without success. He was employed in the meat department of a supermarket, where he experienced considerable *difficulty in maintaining schedules, following directions,* and responding to authority. He also reported *problems following conversations, especially in noisy environments. Spelling and writing tasks* continued to present problems. He noted that he was not yet financially independent, lived at home with his mother, and had *few social contacts.* He stated that his *father evidenced similar problems* and that his *sister was "hyperactive."* Mr. B felt that his *self-esteem was very low* and wanted to remediate some of these limitations in order to improve his social contacts.

Mr. B's medical history included a normal birth history, removal of tonsils and adenoids at age 10, *severe ear infections* beginning in early childhood and which remained to a mild degree, *hyperactivity in childhood*, repair of a deviated septum, and use of corrective lenses. He was currently undergoing visual perceptual training with an ophthalmologist. Hearing and tympanometry were assessed to be normal at the time of CAP testing. Mr. B displayed mildly dysmorphic facial features, a prognathic jaw, and a severe malocclusion. A recent neurological examination ruled out seizures as a causative factor in what was described by Mr. B as his periods of *"tuning out."*

Kevin

Kevin was a 12-year, 4-month-old boy who lived with his father and stepmother and who attended the fifth grade in a regular classroom. He had lived with his mother and half-siblings in another state until recently. He was diagnosed as *learning disabled/dyslexic* in his former school system, where he received resource-room help from the second through current grades. Kevin had been retained in kindergarten.

Recent testing through his present school district identified significant *reading decoding, word identification, and comprehension deficits,* in addition to probable *short-term auditory* and visual *memory difficulties*. A recent Committee of Special Education meeting confirmed the classification of *learning disabled*.

It was suggested to Kevin's parents that outside counseling be sought as a means for him to discuss anger issues. Psychological counseling had just begun when the referral was made to rule out central auditory dysfunction. Kevin's parents had reported *problems with retaining auditory information over time, following directions, and screening out ambient noise distractions*. The psychologist who provided the counseling did not feel that Kevin evidenced *attention deficit disorder,* although a tendency toward *impulsivity* had been noted.

Kevin's father indicated that his son suffered from *chronic ear infections* from birth to age three. Pressure-equalizing tubes had not been inserted. *Speech and language milestones* were *significantly delayed*. Kevin was enrolled in a preschool speech-language therapy program which produced very positive results, according to the father. Other medical history was considered nonsignificant. Visual acuity as reported by the parents was normal. An audiological evaluation indicated normal auditory acuity. However, an examination of brain-stem potentials on the same date indicated *difficulties processing rapid, brief stimuli*.

Kevin indicated ambivalent feelings about school, stating that he did not succeed in any subject and had particular *problems with reading and spelling*. He indicated a keen interest and competency with computers. Kevin stated that *noisy classrooms* make it *difficult for him to concentrate*. He also noted that he *did not sit close to the chalkboard* at this time. Kevin's *self-esteem, in terms of learning, was poor*. Basically good peer interactions were reported by both the classroom teacher and his parents.

Michael

Michael was a 13-year, 1-month-old boy who attended the eighth grade. He was classified as *learning disabled* and received one period of resource-room help daily. While computation math skills were satisfactory, *verbal and logic-oriented tasks presented problems. Reading comprehension* and *language skills were generally weak.* Michael's mother indicated that throughout preschool, kindergarten, and first grade, Michael succeeded academically. In second grade, problems began to surface in the areas of reading and language. Subsequent testing at a local teaching hospital indicated a diagnosis of learning disability and *difficulties with the auditory learning channel* (including *auditory figure-ground problems*). Michael's school system completed testing at the end of fifth grade and came to similar conclusions. Because of continuing social and academic difficulties, the parents requested an evaluation for central auditory processing disorder. Additional testing by a behavioral psychologist ruled out attention deficit disorder.

Michael's mother indicated that early speech-language milestones were normal. He suffered from *moderate ear infections* in early childhood; treatment did not include the insertion of pressure-equalizing tubes. The mother also noted that Michael was born one month overdue, *sustained a 105-degree fever within twelve hours of birth,* and was diagnosed with a calcium deficiency. Other significant medical information included a history of chronic strep infections and a diagnosis of diabetes. An audiological evaluation and tympanometric screening noted normal functioning.

Michael, the elder of two male siblings, had *difficulty maintaining focus* and interest in activities, was artistic, and displayed *pragmatic deficiencies* in his *conversations related to topic choice and maintenance.* Michael's mother felt that he suffered from *low self-esteem* and had poor *peer relationships.*

Sean

Sean was an 11-year, 11-month-old, *left-handed* boy who resided with a younger brother and two parents. He attended the seventh grade, where he received services for *reading difficulties.* Although his *grades had been falling* in the last three years, at the point of the assessment the *school district had not labeled him in any way.* Sean's mother reported that one of his former teachers raised the issue of attention deficit disorder due to the symptoms of *distractibility, impulsivity, lack of focus, and disorganization* within the classroom. Sean's current teachers reported similar behaviors and *improved performance in one-to-one contexts.* Sean generally liked school, where he enjoyed reading and spelling and disliked social studies and math. A diagnosis of attention deficit disorder was ruled out after testing by a behavioral psychologist. However, due to observations made during testing and behaviors reported by Sean's parents, such as *difficulty in following directions* and *distractibility in noise,* the referral was made to rule out central auditory processing dysfunction.

The mother also reported that low-powered reading glasses were recently recommended for Sean. He suffered from severe allergies and was a chronic open-mouth breather. Sean also suffered from *ear infections in infancy and early childhood,* but, according to his mother, not chronically. Other medical history reported by the mother was considered nonsignificant. His mother noted poor socialization skills, *poor coordination, social immaturity,* generally adequate self-esteem, and exceptional skill in playing the tuba. An audiological evaluation indicated he was within normal limits of functioning.

Brendan

Brendan was an *energetic* three-year-old boy who attended preschool. He had been identified as *"speech impaired"* and received speech-language services twice weekly for *phonological disorder*. Recent testing through his school district, however, suggested a change in label to *attention deficit hyperactivity disorder*. Brendan's mother reported that significant behavior problems had been identified by the preschool. Additional problems noted by his mother included *frequent screaming at home, poor peer relationships, highly destructible behaviors, inability to follow directions (especially in noise) and hypersensitivity to noise*.

Brendan experienced *frequent ear infections* from approximately six months through 18 months of age. Pressure-equalizing tubes were inserted and had since fallen out. No current infections had been noted. Pure-tone testing could not be completed because of behavior; however, Brendan's ability to repeat SRT words at 15 db. suggested to the audiologist that hearing was within the speech range. Tympanometric testing indicated normal middle-ear functioning. Further pure-tone testing was strongly recommended. Brendan's mother reported additional medical history that was considered nonsignificant. She also noted that although Brendan's first words occurred at approximately one year of age, *subsequent expressive and receptive language milestones appeared delayed*.

Brendan's mother sought psychological counseling for the purpose of alleviating some of the behavior problems. She felt strongly that behavior issues were paramount and that she needed guidance in terms of intervention strategies. A referral was then made to clarify suspected central auditory processing difficulties.

Jeffrey

Jeffrey was a pleasant 12-year-old boy who attended seventh grade in a regular junior high school. He lived with his mother and six siblings. The mother reported normal developmental milestones for speech and language and a nonsignificant medical history. Jeffrey had experienced *academic problems* since kindergarten. According to the mother, the school district had performed tests at various times since kindergarten, but had not specifically labeled Jeffrey. However, *resource-room services* were made available to him as needed. Jeffrey had significant *difficulties with following directions and phonics,* as well as with *writing and spelling activities*. Problems within the classroom appeared both academic and *attentional*. He was either *failing or barely passing all of his subjects*. Teachers had reported *poor attitude and effort* in addition to *"tuning out"* behaviors. Jeffrey had been *acting out in the classroom* and cutting numerous classes. Jeffrey reported that he noticed problems in *focusing, following directions, and dealing with background noises*. Just prior to the CAP evaluation, Jeffrey had been tested privately by a psychologist associated with a local university. Intellectual skills were found to be within normal limits, and visual processing skills were found to be strong. Audiological testing revealed normal functioning. At the point of CAP testing, Jeffrey's *self-esteem was extremely low* and he appeared *very frustrated*.

Lori

Lori was a personable seven-year-old girl who was the younger of two siblings within an intact family. She was a second grader who received *resource-room help* one hour daily, *primarily for reading decoding and comprehension problems*. Teachers had reported problems with *impulsivity, distractibility, completion of tasks, and academic difficulties with reading and spelling*. Lori was tested by the school psychologist and was determined to evidence *attention deficit hyperactivity disorder*. Findings included a determination of 100 performance and 88 verbal I.Q. levels. Lori was taking Ritalin (twice daily) for use in school only. The mother felt that only minimal gains were made in school in terms of Lori's difficulties. It was recommended to the parents to seek additional testing to further clarify Lori's learning profile. The mother reported that Lori had difficulties in *following directions, especially in the presence of background noise*. She also stated that Lori had *poor peer relationships, did not like group activities, and had problems completing deferred directions*. According to Lori, she had greater difficulties comprehending in *noisy environments*. She also indicated that she *"hated" spelling and language* but "loved" math.

A nonsignificant medical history was reported. The mother noted that Lori had only two ear infections to date. An audiological evaluation indicated normal hearing acuity.

Otitis Media

Many factors in a child's medical, educational, and psychosocial background are important to identify when assessing CAPD. One of these factors, otitis media, although not clearly causative in terms of processing disorders, appears to be at least associative.

Otitis media can be a serious health concern that necessitates early identification and treatment in children. According to the National Center for Health Statistics, it is the most common illness in children between birth and three years of age. Otitis media with effusion is an inflammation of the middle ear which may result in permanent or transient hearing loss. Acute otitis media is a condition in which the symptoms last approximately three weeks. When the middle-ear effusion lasts more than three months, it is considered chronic otitis media. Recurrent otitis media implies repeated infections of the middle ear, perhaps four to five incidences over a 6- to 12-month period.

Nonsurgical management typically involves antimicrobial agents such as ampicillin, sulfonamide, or erythromycin. The most common surgical treatment is myringotomy with insertion of tympanostomy or pressure-equalizing tubes in the eardrum. The earlier the age of the first incidence of otitis media, the greater the probability of subsequent significant occurrence (Howie et al. 1975; Paradise 1980; Shurin et al. 1979). Fluid within the middle-ear cavity may remain for weeks or months after treatment (Klein 1983). Considering the fact that retained fluid may remain for extended periods of time after treatment and that many children suffer from recurrent episodes, the concerns about hearing sensitivity in these children is great, especially during the critical language learning period of birth to age three (Lenneberg 1967).

In early infancy, children discriminate speech sounds in their environment. They begin to correlate a developing sound system with linguistic rules. Inconsistent auditory stimuli may create confusion in the child who is trying to acquire word meanings and grammatical rules (Berko-Gleason 1983).

Numerous studies have focused on the effects (or absence of effects) of otitis media on various aspects of children's language development, auditory processing, and later school performance. While some studies maintain a negative impact upon development and/or performance, others disagree. Few studies have examined specific aspects of central auditory processing and language performance. A brief summary of several significant studies centering upon various aspects of language will follow (see pages 22-23).

However, at this point, we will examine possible reasons for the controversy in the literature.

Ventry (1980) reviewed published research that focused on the relationship between conductive hearing loss and language learning problems. He concluded that the inconsistencies in findings might be due to poor research design. Variables such as age, intelligence, sex, socioeconomic status, race, grade level, and other illnesses might account for group differences. Additionally, subject selection and hearing loss at the time of administration of the research task also may impact upon performance. Ventry also noted poorly calibrated instruments, inappropriate tests, and researcher bias as other possible factors.

Allen and Robinson (1984) offered additional insight into the lack of definitive information between middle-ear dysfunction and language performance. The existence and duration of episodes of middle-ear disease are difficult to document, especially because effusion is often asymptomatic. Also, it is difficult to quantify hearing loss in very young children due to testing limitations.

The lack of specific criteria to classify "chronic" otitis media is also problematic. In some settings "chronic" may imply any incidence beyond two episodes per year, while other settings may take a more conservative view.

While chronic otitis media may negatively impact on development or performance, recurrent acute otitis media may not present any problem. Definitive identification and documentation is often lacking in the research. Additionally, some studies appear to lack specific identification of the particular language skill examined. Perhaps more studies should be narrowly focused to examine individual aspects of language (for example, receptive vocabulary, auditory memory, and others) rather than to examine broader parameters.

Also complicating analysis is the fact that research data may be interpreted from various perspectives. For example, one can assume an indirect relationship between otitis media accompanied by mild, fluctuating hearing loss and language mediated by hearing. One could also assume that the relationship between otitis media, hearing, and language may change over time. Friel-Patti (1990) maintained that the relationship between otitis media and language development is indirect, remediated by hearing, and changeable over time. Some children may evidence negative effects from otitis media while passing through the critical language acquisition stage, but may remediate on their own as they get older.

Ellenmorris Tiegerman, Ph.D., commented upon the relationship between chronic otitis media and language development in preschool children with language impairment (Kelly 1993a). She maintained that an association existed between otitis media and pervasive language dysfunction. According to Tiegerman, otitis media may exacerbate an already existing problem, creating language learning problems due to information that is episodic and erratic (Kelly 1993a). Thus, another issue comes to light. Studies often cannot verify that subjects would have been "language normal" in the absence of otitis media.

Another crucial flaw in studies completed in this area is that many of them are retrospective in nature. Subjects are frequently chosen on the basis of language and academic problems. Histories are examined to explain the causes for these problems. A preferred method would be to study a group of children over time until the points at which developmental difficulties may be expected (Friel-Patti 1990).

Harold Levinson, M.D., studied approximately 25,000 cases of dyslexia and commented upon the relationship between ear infections and speech-language impairments (Kelly 1993b). While age of onset and chronicity are important factors, the more critical problems arise when the infections cause inner-ear nerve damage. Levinson maintained that delays in speech-language development should not be examined in terms of hearing loss alone.

According to Boone (1987, 165), children who experience otitis media over several years are more likely to demonstrate auditory comprehension problems even after the infections have ceased. Children's listening skills may be affected by hearing loss in the preschool years. In many children classified as learning disabled, prior hearing loss may have been a primary cause for comprehension problems (Boone 1987, 165).

A brief recounting of some recent studies and publications focusing upon otitis media and various aspects of language performance follows. Among those which found a correlation between histories of otitis media and various aspects of language development are these:

1. Gravel and Wallace (1992) found that otitis-positive four-year-old children needed a more advantageous signal-to-competition ratio for sentence intelligibility when compared to otitis-negative peers.

2. Friel-Patti and Finitzo (1990) studied otitis media with effusion during the first two years of life and noted that better language was associated with better hearing levels. The relationship between otitis media and language development may be indirectly affected by hearing and may improve over time.

3. Zinkus (1986) studied the relationship between otitis media, conductive hearing loss, and speech, language, and academic skills. He found positive correlations between hearing loss (even when only slight to moderate) and delayed performance.

4. Scaldwell (1985), studying otitis media in Cree and Ojibway children four to 16 years old, found a high incidence of otitis media in those who had language impairment.

5. Reichman and Healey (1983) reviewed the research on the relationship between otitis media and learning/language/hearing disorders and found that the incidence of otitis media was double in learning-disabled as opposed to nonlearning-disabled children.

6. Quick and Mandell (1983) studied the relationship between middle-ear fluid (with conductive hearing loss) and learning disabilities, and found that potential effects may include auditory processing deficits and generalized speech and language deficits.

Other studies and publications indicate a negative correlation between a history of otitis media and various aspects of language performance.

1. For two years, Paul et al. (1993) studied toddlers (normally speaking and late-talking, with and without positive histories of otitis media). They found no differences in expressive language outcomes; however, differences in articulation performances were discovered.

2. Grievink et al. (1993) examined the relationship between early otitis media with effusion (OME) and later language abilities in children with bilateral OME. Even up to nine instances of OME, intermittent or continuous, did not negatively affect language to age seven.

3. Roberts et al. (1991) studied the effects of early otitis media with effusion and later language development in children from both lower- and middle-income families and found no reliable relationship.

4. Roberts et al. (1988) examined the relationship between otitis media in early childhood and the number of common phonological processes or consonants in error noted in 55 socioeconomically disadvantaged children. No significant relationship was found. However, otitis media in early childhood was associated with the total number of phonological processes evidenced between ages 4 and 6 years, 8 months.

5. Allen and Robinson (1984) studied 602 preschool children and found no consistent relationship between middle-ear status as judged by impedance screening and language development as assessed by performance on a standardized language measure.

6. A retrospective study found that children with positive histories of OME had greater difficulty recognizing monosyllabic words than their OME-negative peers (Jerger et al. 1983).

7. Menyuk (1980) stated that available evidence did not support a positive relationship between otitis media in infancy and the preschool years and later language and academic performance.

8. Children with a history of chronic otitis media seem to have more severe difficulties in central auditory processing skills such as auditory sequential memory, sound blending, and auditory discrimination than children who had simple auditory processing deficits (Gottlieb and Zinkus 1980),

Interestingly, a recent survey released by the American Academy of Pediatrics (Physician Survey 1994) indicated that 65% of physicians polled believed that middle-ear infections can impair language. Additionally, 83% believed that ear infections can cause temporary hearing loss, and 46.7% believed that infections could result in permanent hearing loss.

In sum, it appears that the controversy surrounding the effects of otitis media upon language development is as yet unresolved. However, speech-language pathologists should be aware of a condition known as minimal auditory deficiency syndrome, which has been defined by Martin (1986, 337) as "changes in the size of neurons in the central nervous system caused by conductive-hearing loss in early life. The result is difficulty in language learning." In effect, even temporary and mild conductive-hearing losses, commonly associated with chronic otitis media, may negatively affect the skills needed for language learning. Skinner (1978, 311-327) has identified as many as eight factors which can negatively affect language development in the young child who experiences erratic auditory input. Therefore, it appears advantageous for the speech-language pathologist to be fully aware of possible effects of chronic otitis media and to approach intervention from the perspective of possible early sensory deprivation and subsequent skill limitations.

CAPDs and Learning Disabilities, Attention Deficit Disorder, and Dyslexia

Central auditory processing disorders may exist as either primary or secondary disorders. Specifically, CAPD can be the only identifiable condition in an individual or can be viewed in relationship to a more basic condition such as learning disabilities or attention deficit disorder. This is not to imply that all children who have learning disabilities, attention deficit disorder, or dyslexia necessarily also evidence central auditory processing disorders. The following chart depicts the possible relationships among the various conditions.

Primary Diagnosis	Secondary Diagnosis
CAPD	
LD	CAPD
ADD	CAPD
Dyslexia	CAPD

Learning disabilities, attention deficit disorder, and dyslexia may exist in various combinations within any individual. For example, a very common combination is learning disabilities with attention deficit disorder. For clarity, when CAPD is the primary diagnosis, perhaps the term *specific central auditory processing disorder (SCAPD)* would be appropriate. This term would indicate that the disorder does not apparently coexist with other conditions such as learning disabilities or attention deficit disorder or dyslexia.

We will not attempt here to provide extensive information regarding learning disabilities, attention deficit disorder, or dyslexia. Rather, we will identify their possible interactions and reiterate their common features. The following listing of characteristics suggests a possible common underlying mechanism pervasive to all four conditions (and possibly to others such as cluttering and childhood aphasia). A somewhat similar concept centering upon dyslexia has been described by psychiatrist/author Harold Levinson, M.D. (Kelly 1993b). This notion also suggests a possible higher-order auditory dysfunction in some cases.

It is advantageous for the speech-language pathologist to view such conditions broadly, noting possible social, psychological, behavioral, academic, and medical issues. These characteristics will be present to varying degrees in any particular individual and may be absent in others.

Children who have auditory-visual integration difficulties may perform well on tasks that are purely auditory *or* visual, but fail when the tasks are combined. For example, some children perform well on auditory discrimination tests based only on auditory stimuli and fail when tests involve the selection of pictures.

	CAPD	LD	ADD	Dyslexia
Hyperactivity		✔	✔	
Attention deficits	✔	✔	✔	✔
Language deficits	✔	✔	✔	✔
Motor deficits				
Concept development deficits	✔	✔	✔	✔
Impulsivity		✔	✔	
Memory deficits	✔	✔	✔	✔
Spatial relationship deficits		✔	✔	✔
Temporal relationship deficits	✔	✔	✔	✔
Reading deficits	✔	✔	✔	✔
Writing deficits	✔	✔	✔	✔
Math deficits		✔	✔	
Articulation/phonology deficits	✔	✔	✔	✔
Pragmatic deficits	✔	✔	✔	
Low frustration tolerance	✔	✔	✔	
Low self-esteem	✔	✔	✔	✔
Disorganization	✔	✔	✔	
Related family history	✔	✔	✔	✔
Poor social relationships	✔	✔	✔	✔
Difficulty with logic	✔	✔	✔	

The observation of subnormal musical skills may be possible as well. Deficiency may be relevant if a lack of prosody in the child's oral expressions also has been observed. Therapy in this case may involve development of rhythm, rate, pitch, and volume changes.

These characteristics may be extracted into fundamental, although abbreviated, definitions of learning disabilities, attention deficit disorder, and dyslexia:

- *Learning disabilities*—Disorders in one or more of the basic psychological processes involved in the understanding or use of spoken or written language. May be evidenced as difficulties in listening, speaking, reading, writing, spelling, math, and other areas. Some may be associated with specific preschool children with language impairment who demonstrate qualitative differences in auditory process functioning.

- *Attention deficit disorder*—A disorder frequently involving inattentiveness and distractibility, overarousal, impulsivity, difficulty with gratification, visual and/or auditory processing disorders, and other characteristics. May or may not involve hyperactivity and/or social, language, and academic problems.

  Children with attention deficit disorder should be differentiated from children with executive dysfunction (EDF). While both groups share some common characteristics, they differ in terms of basis. Both groups may have difficulty completing tasks. However, while the typical ADD child is unable to focus or maintain attention, the EDF child is unable to self-regulate, is unorganized, and is unable to move from one task to another without redirection. The EDF child may not know how to break down the task into manageable components or how to get started. The EDF child differs from the ADD child in that the former condition appears more cognitively based, while the latter condition appears more attentionally based.

- *Dyslexia*—A failure to master reading at expected age levels. May also involve writing, spelling, math, speech, language, attentional difficulties, and other problems. Can be subgrouped into auditory, visual, and auditory-visual categories.

PART TWO

Diagnosis

Part Two is designed to apply the more generalized information offered in Part One in a practical, clinical manner.

Chapter 2, Foundations for Diagnosis, provides information concerning the assessment process, describes criteria for candidacy, and lists various assessment tools.

Chapter 3, Diagnostic Specifics, provides detailed and specific materials for the diagnostic process, including checklists, a case history form, and a report format.

2
Foundations for Diagnosis

Diagnosis

Children with central auditory processing disorder are diagnosed primarily by the speech-language pathologist and the audiologist. Each discipline has particular theoretical approaches, protocols, and expertises in both diagnosis and intervention. Both professionals pool information on an ongoing and cooperative basis. Within the school setting, the Committee of Special Education (C.S.E.), or whatever counterpart has been indicated, ultimately confirms the diagnosis and makes recommendations regarding placement and services.

Referrals for diagnostic evaluations may be made through several channels, including psychologists, parents, physicians, school nurses, classroom teachers, and reading teachers.

The speech-language pathologist often indicates the need for assessment based on classroom observations. This is particularly likely within the last few years because many therapists now are based in the classroom rather than in the therapy room. The school may specify a protocol for referrals rather than leaving the process largely to chance. A protocol may require the speech-language pathologist to periodically screen children who are at risk. The procedure also may require speech-language pathologists to identify and explain various factors of CAPD to teachers.

Intervention

Intervention, particularly within the school system, is usually the responsibility of the speech-language pathologist, although ongoing consultation with the psychologist, classroom teacher, resource room teacher, nurse, and other team members is very important. The child with CAPD must be treated as a "whole" child with a variety of characteristics and concerns and not be considered the sole clinical responsibility of the speech-language pathologist.

Intervention also involves continual input from the audiologist regarding hearing status, especially when chronic otitis media is an issue. The audiologist is also needed when an assistive listening device or auditory trainer is used. The audiologist recommends the most appropriate unit, adjusts it to the child's particular audiological needs, and maintains it mechanically.

Support Teams

Support team members include all persons involved with treatment of the child with CAPD. Members of the team may include the classroom teacher, special education teacher, resource-room teacher, reading teacher, nurse, physician, psychologist, audiologist, social worker, parent, speech-language pathologist, and the child. Occasionally, the input of other professionals (such as the teacher of English as a Second Language) is indicated. Support team members will have varying degrees of involvement; however, intervention clearly is a group effort, and perspectives from a variety of viewpoints are helpful.

Perhaps the most important perspective is that which comes from the child. *How a child experiences CAPD*—that is, how it impacts on the child's life in specific ways—is critical. When we can identify the most difficult areas from the child's perspective, we can better key into motivational factors. For example, a child may feel motivated to improve auditory discrimination skills in order to follow conversations better on the playground, while we may want to improve similar skills for spelling or reading decoding purposes. Clearly, it is ideal when both interests can be combined. Make the child a vital participant in the intervention process. The process of growth should not happen "to" the child, but "with" the child.

Issues Related to Assessment

Probably the most significant problem in central auditory processing assessment is knowing exactly what is being assessed. Factors such as linguistic skills (particularly vocabulary levels), attention, cognitive ability, and attitude or effort can all affect test results. For example, is the child scoring poorly on an auditory memory test because of deficient memory, or because of problems related to attention or vocabulary? Separating the central auditory processing factors from other possible influences is often difficult.

The test environment itself may be inappropriate. For example, if the tests are being taken in a school where there is considerable hallway noise, auditory figure-ground deficits may affect the test results. Test settings that contain many visual distractions may impair performance in a child with visual figure-ground difficulties. The child may evidence other problems that are unrelated to auditory processing. These problems must be considered when completing an assessment.

Another potential hazard concerns hearing sensitivity. Although a full audiological evaluation and tympanometric screening (indicating middle-ear status) should precede central auditory processing testing, in some cases (especially in children with histories of otitis media), hearing levels may change between the audiological evaluation and the CAP assessment. To avoid this, both assessments should be completed on the same day if the child can maintain attention. Otherwise, the assessments may be separated by a single day or two.

Another issue arises concerning the hearing sensitivity levels of children with chronic histories of otitis media. Audiological testing is typically completed when the child is infection-free. However, it is more helpful to have sensitivity information from at least two points: when a typical infection is in full force as well as when the child is infection-free. If the child suffers from chronic infections in which a loss of hearing sensitivity is suspected, it would be helpful to know about hearing status during these frequent periods in the child's life. During these "abnormal" periods, perception and processing may be at risk. These periods, particularly in the critical language-learning years, may contribute to some processing problems. Testing may be time-consuming, costly, and difficult to complete in some cases; but for this purpose, even basic screening information would be beneficial. Tympanometric information also should be available regularly and frequently.

Selection of assessment tools is important in terms of identifying all possible areas of disorder. The assessment tools should be norm-referenced whenever possible.

A variety of high- and low-structured procedures also should be selected so that skills may be viewed from more than one perspective. The specific protocols that are provided in this book are meant to be representative plans of assessment. No one single protocol may be considered problem-free and clinically perfect.

How a child takes a test and *how* the child fails a particular task is often very telling in terms of central auditory processing disorder. For example, at what point in the auditory memory sentence test did the child begin to fail? Did the child seem to recall beginning and end units and miss the middle ones? Patterns that emerge may be helpful when planning intervention strategies.

Another clinical issue centers on interpretation of results. It is not enough in CAPD testing to simply report results and diagnose exclusively in terms of deficient scores. Since CAPDs are multifaceted, often impacting upon academic, linguistic, and social performances, "relationships" between particular test results and problem areas (such as spelling or inability to follow directions at home) must be identified. These evaluations may be thought of as puzzles that often provide answers to troubling questions and provide insight into patterns of behavior. Sometimes the diagnosis itself provides a degree of relief to frustrated and confused parents and students.

The question of whether the speech-language assessment protocol for CAPD tests language or auditory processing is complex and may never be resolved definitively. However, the protocols which are provided in this book have been selected with this issue in mind. Assessment tools and procedures are identified that examine key representative aspects of language functioning as well as auditory processing skills. The importance of possible effects of deficient auditory processing skills on language performance is recognized and addressed. In addition to a full audiological evaluation and tympanometric screening, a more typical speech-language evaluation should precede the CAPD battery in order to examine language performance in detail.

Approaches to Diagnosis

Central auditory processing assessment may be approached from several perspectives, two of which are the most relevant for purposes of this book. The speech-language pathologist generally identifies disorders of processing in terms of language abilities and language-dependent behaviors. The audiologist typically views processing disorders as breakdowns in the functioning of the auditory nervous system. Controls over language influences and other nonauditory factors such as cognitive ability and attention are important in such testing. In reality, however, it may be impossible to completely separate auditory processing skills from language and behavior. Matkin and Hook (1983, 226) differentiate these approaches and their respective assessment procedures as the Central Auditory Function Battery (as per the language-learning specialist) and the Central Audiologic Battery (as per the audiologist).

Typically, lesions that are based in the outer or middle ears, the sensory cells of the cochlea, or the auditory nerve result in loss of hearing sensitivity and are largely measurable using pure tones (the test-battery approach). These lesions tend to be easier to diagnose than lesions at the level of the olivary complex and beyond. The latter condition tends to produce apparent hearing symptoms in the ears ipsilateral to the lesions; while in the former condition, because both sides of the brain are involved in the transmission of auditory information, diagnosis is difficult. Audiological symptoms may be nonexistent or very mild. Audiologists, therefore, have discovered that conventional testing measures, including use of pure tones and masking, often are disappointing for purposes of identifying these central auditory lesions.

Generally, while site-of-lesion testing is helpful for the peripheral areas of the auditory pathways (cochlear nuclei and auditory nerve), such testing cannot identify pathology in higher centers. There exists an additional caution with regard to possible overreliance on site-of-lesion batteries. In patients with both a cochlear and central auditory disorder, most audiological tests will reflect only the outermost or most peripheral lesion. Because one lesion has been identified, it is not necessarily true that it is the only lesion.

Because the use of pure-tone audiometry has been of minimal use, audiologists often use speech-based tests as part of a battery. The vocabulary levels of such tests should be low enough so that if a young child has difficulty, failure can be reasonably attributed to a central auditory processing disorder rather than to a vocabulary problem.

Jerger and Jerger (1971) described the use of the performance-intensity function of phonetically balanced (PB) words as a viable means of screening for central auditory disorders. Other procedures used for diagnosis include Binaural Fusion (Willeford 1977), Low-Pass Filtered Speech (Willeford 1977), Staggered Spondaic Word Test (SSW, Katz 1968), Competing Sentences Test (Willeford 1977), Pitch Pattern Test (Pinheiro 1977), Rapidly Alternating Speech Perception Test (Willeford 1977), and Competing Environmental Sounds Test (Katz 1977), among others.

Auditory brainstem response audiometry is beneficial in diagnosing central auditory disorders in cases where hearing loss exists which is basically mild and equal in both ears. Recent attempts to manipulate the auditory signal in terms of time appear to be very promising.

The neurologist also may diagnose central auditory processing disorders. Examination may rely upon tests such as the electroencephalogram, CT scan, Positron Emission Tomography, arteriogram, assessment of regional cerebral blood flow, or spinal tap. A detailed developmental history is taken, including information regarding fetal movements and possible seizures. A thorough physical examination is completed, with close attention paid to growth progress and head size.

The psychiatrist or psychologist also may diagnose CAPD through psychological testing. In most cases, the profile which may reveal a pattern is more important than the individual scores. Perceptual modes of learning and communication styles are determined, and social and emotional adaptations and accompanying behavior disorders are noted. Levels of cognitive functioning, including problem-solving strategies, are observed.

Speech-language pathologists generally assume a different approach in assessment of individuals with CAPD. Attempts are made to examine language functioning and the possible effects of central auditory processing disorder on language-dependent behaviors. A truly comprehensive diagnosis may involve input from a variety of sources.

Screening and Diagnostic Evaluations

Screening procedures are never designed to replace full diagnostic evaluations, especially in the case of a child with central auditory processing disorder. The procedures have two very different purposes. The screening procedure attempts to rule out the more gross or general areas of central auditory processing dysfunction in a child who may be at risk, or as a precautionary or early identification process with the so-called normal child (kindergartner). This process, when coupled with tympanometric and audiological screenings, usually is effective.

Several commercially produced screening tools assess one or more aspects of possible dysfunction. It would appear more advantageous to compile a screening protocol that can observe a variety of key skill areas (for example, auditory memory and auditory figure-ground skills) rather than to simply examine one or two. The informal screening plan that follows (pages 34-35) is merely suggestive and is designed to briefly examine all key skill areas. It is meant to be combined with audiological and tympanometric procedures. Depending upon site limitations and numbers of children involved, you may also wish to use other observational tools, such as the ones designed for teacher and parent use.

The diagnostic evaluation is meant to clarify in considerable detail the specific nature of central auditory processing disorder. It can be accomplished only on a one-to-one basis and involves a full battery of assessment tools. This battery is completed on children who have failed screening procedures or otherwise present cause for diagnosis (for example, psychologist or pediatrician recommendation). A full audiological evaluation and tympanometric screening are necessary prerequisites to this type of testing. Detailed information about speech and language functioning also is important. Protocols for full diagnostic evaluations for central auditory processing disorder will follow (pages 38-41).

Child's Name:	Grade/Placement:
Speech-Language Pathologist:	Date:

Reason for Screening:

Screening for Central Auditory Processing Disorder

Skill Area I: Auditory Memory

Assessment Tool: Test of Auditory Perceptual Skills	Results:	Status:
Auditory Number Memory Forward:		
Auditory Sentence Memory:		

Skill Area II: Auditory Discrimination

Assessment Tool: Test of Auditory Perceptual Skills	Results:	Status:
Auditory Word Discrimination; or		
Test of Language Development-P Word Discrimination (subtest)		

Skill Area III: Auditory Figure-Ground

Assessment Tool: Goldman-Fristoe-Woodcock *Test of Auditory Discrimination,*	Results:	Status:
Noise Subtest		

(continued)

Central Auditory Processing Disorder / Dorothy A. Kelly, D.A. / ISBN 0761631623

Skill Area IV: Auditory Cohesion

Assessment Tool: Test of Auditory Perceptual Skills Auditory Processing (thinking and reasoning)	Results:	Status:

Skill Area V: Auditory Attention

Assessment Tool: Clinical/Informant Observations:	Results:	Status:

Summary:

Recommendations:

_____
Speech-Language Pathologist

Central Auditory Processing Disorder / Dorothy A. Kelly, D.A. / ISBN 0761631623

Early Identification of CAPD in Preschool or Kindergarten

There are a significant number of elementary school-age children with either primary or secondary central auditory processing disorder. Some of these children demonstrate symptoms of CAPD secondarily to a primary disorder such as learning disabilities or attention deficit disorder. Often the central auditory processing component to the profile is overlooked or described by other labels. These children frequently exhibit a wide variety of attentional and behavioral difficulties and often demonstrate problems with reading, spelling, speaking, following directions, expressive language, and vocabulary, among other areas. Many develop poor self-esteem and negative attitudes about school. The emotional behavioral effects may be largely preventable through early identification of CAPD symptoms.

More broadly based screening procedures of central auditory processing disorders would prove cost-effective to school districts in the long run. This is not to imply that with early intervention, "miracle cures" are possible. Rather, with early identification, children with CAPDs may be provided with strategies and skills to facilitate greater academic and language success. Success often directly translates into improved self-esteem, especially when efforts are coordinated both at school and at home.

Preschool or (at the very latest) kindergarten programs could screen the following areas with minimal effort: auditory figure-ground, ability to follow one- and two-step commands, delayed auditory recall of a simple nonsense word (after 10 minutes), auditory discrimination with a visual component (choosing one picture from a field of four), and receptive vocabulary. Information about hearing acuity and tympanometric status also is important.

This type of approach is proactive rather than reactive. It focuses on all children as potential candidates for intervention, rather than dealing with children who have already experienced failure in some way. It also would be helpful to the classroom teacher who then would have information and tools to deal with the child with CAPD from the onset, thus avoiding many frustrations and failures. With early intervention, many cases of CAPD are far less complicated, more manageable, and more remediable, as compared to the multifaceted profiles that develop over time.

Criteria and Candidacy

Central auditory processing disorders take a variety of forms and can range from mild to severe. They may be the primary diagnosis in one individual and the secondary diagnosis in another (for example, as after a stroke). When are the symptoms significant enough that the individual is considered to have central auditory processing disorder? In reality, within the so-called normal population there are varying skill levels. Furthermore, once an individual is diagnosed as having CAPD, does that necessarily imply that he or she is a candidate for therapy?

Whenever at least one aspect of central auditory processing has been verified as below within-normal limits (WNL) of functioning, the individual should then be considered central auditory processing impaired. This label does not specify degree or range, but simply indicates that at least an aspect of disorder is present. It is not a label of prognosis, only of diagnosis, and it should be specified further as a primary or secondary condition and described in terms of severity.

With regard to candidacy for therapy, most school systems stipulate that the impairment must be significant enough to interfere with academic functioning as evidenced by poor grades. Hypothetically, children with milder degrees of disorder in perhaps one or two of the main skill areas might "fall through the cracks" and never be identified or tested. These children have probably learned coping strategies on their own that allowed them to "just get by." Many of these children suffer from mild problems in auditory memory, figure-ground, and/or auditory cohesion.

Conversely, there could be a child who demonstrates minimal or no processing disorder symptoms in school and who attains grade-level performance or better, but in reality has specific deficits (for example, auditory figure-ground) which appear mainly at home. Perhaps the child's classroom setting is highly structured and relatively quiet, while the home setting is not. This is an instance where an evaluation of the "whole child" becomes all the more important. This also is a child who may "fall through the cracks." Because the child is doing well academically, and because the deficit is narrowly defined and mild in degree, typical school systems would not consider this child a candidate for therapy. An option for this child's parents would be to obtain services from a private practitioner and to modify the listening environment at home as much as possible.

CAPD is often a secondary diagnosis present within populations with conditions such as learning disabilities and attention deficit disorder. Members of the latter groups are often placed within self-contained or resource-room settings where supportive services may include speech-language pathology. Such children minimally should be screened for CAPD. If CAPD proves to be an integral part of the child's learning profile, then such "root" issues should be addressed. For example, the auditory discrimination problems of a child with learning disability certainly impact negatively on reading and spelling skills. This is not to imply that all children with LD or ADD have problems in central auditory processing; however, many of them do. Wouldn't it be advantageous to screen all members of the self-contained classroom for CAPD, regardless of whether they presently receive speech-language services?

It may well be cost effective in the long run to screen all children within the typical kindergarten or early intervention settings. Through early identification of disorder, would it not be possible to "prevent" (or at least reduce in severity) subsequent academic failure? In this case, candidacy would not be based upon already demonstrated academic failure as much as a recognition of "red alert" factors in advance.

Many school systems now recognize "fluctuating hearing loss" (that is, as per otitis media) as a basis for speech-language services if the condition has impacted negatively on classroom performance. This enlightened policy recognizes that in many cases a fluctuating or inconsistent auditory signal can be more devastating to a child than a mild or even moderate permanent hearing loss. It is often the inconsistency of the auditory experience that proves most destructive. Other children who do not have a present and ongoing history of otitis media also may "fall through the cracks." The damage has already been done in some cases; the previous history of otitis media may have had a negative impact (for example, auditory discrimination or figure-ground problems). If the deficits are mild or do not significantly impact on academic performance, they are not likely to be identified.

In general, some degree of CAPD testing should be integral to all reading and special education inventories. Candidacy should be determined individually, depending upon input from various team members, including parents. Each child's profile is different, and candidacy cannot be determined purely from test scores or classroom grades. For example, a one-year delay in auditory discrimination skills for one child may have minimal academic and social effects, while in another it might prove devastating. In the case of CAPD, prevention, early identification, and flexible candidacy criteria go a long way.

The Diagnostic Evaluation Process: Representative Assessment Tools

The specific assessment tools identified in this book represent a variety of procedures which are selected based on individual profiles, needs, settings, and other factors. For consistency and clarity, a single protocol has been identified in the various profiles and summaries. The two assessment listings below (one for a child and one for an adult) represent some additional choices.

Certain tests seem to have limitations in terms of normative data (that is, the norms are not current) and content of the tasks involved (for example, Is this task testing basic knowledge or auditory reasoning skills?). Appropriate assessment choices must be made. Examination of the various auditory processing skill areas (as identified in Chapter 1) is what is most important. This may be accomplished in a variety of ways. Results from any procedure can be checked through additional procedures (for example, verify figure-ground or auditory memory difficulties with the teacher's and parent's observation checklists).

All protocols should include a case history, full audiological evaluation, additional speech-language testing as indicated, parent and teacher observation forms, reading decoding procedures, spelling procedures, a language sample, an articulation/phonology procedure, a deferred or delayed auditory memory procedure, and other appropriate informal procedures. For guidance in completing these procedures, see Graded Reading Word Lists (pages 49-51), Analysis of Spelling Skills (pages 52-54), and other aids offered in this book. Also refer to the sample diagnostic evaluations (pages 56-80).

It is important to incorporate informally based assessment procedures into any protocol. These procedures often demonstrate how the child performs under more naturalistic circumstances and may provide additional means of "checking" results obtained with formal tests. If the child tires or if attention wanes, testing should be discontinued temporarily. One always wants to be certain of what is being tested. For example, does the child actually have a poor auditory memory, or is the child simply tired or bored?

Auditory Memory

Test of Auditory Perceptual Skills

Screening Test for Auditory Perception

Auditory Memory Span Test

Auditory Sequential Memory Test

Goldman-Fristoe-Woodcock Auditory Memory Tests

Detroit Tests of Learning Aptitude

Test of Language Development—Primary

Carow Auditory-Visual Abilities Test

Wechsler Intelligence Tests for Children—Revised

Illinois Test of Psycholinguistic Abilities—Revised

Woodcock-Johnson Psychoeducational Battery

Survey of Early Childhood Abilities

Language Structured Auditory Retention Span

Test of Memory and Learning

Auditory Discrimination

Test of Language Development—Primary

Wepman Auditory Discrimination Test

Test of Auditory Perceptual Skills

Goldman-Fristoe-Woodcock Test of Auditory Discrimination

SCAN: A Screening Test for Auditory Processing Disorders

Bankson Language Screening Test

Goldman-Fristoe-Woodcock Auditory Skills Test Battery

Survey of Early Childhood Abilities

Auditory Figure-Ground (and/or auditory selection attention)

Goldman-Fristoe-Woodcock Test of Auditory Discrimination, Noise Subtest

SCAN: A Screening Test for Auditory Processing Disorders

Goldman-Fristoe-Woodcock Auditory Skills Test Battery

Auditory Cohesion (as defined in this book)

Test of Auditory Perceptual Skills

Test of Auditory Reasoning and Processing Skills

Survey of Early Childhood Abilities

Test of Memory and Learning

Auditory Attention

Quick Neurological Screening Test—Revised

SCAN: A Screening Test for Auditory Processing Disorders

Auditory Continuous Performance Test

Auditory Perception (as described in this book)

Diagnostic Spelling Potential Test

Test of Auditory Analysis Skills

Test of Kindergarten/First Grade Readiness Skills

Diagnostic Screening Test: Reading

Illinois Test of Psycholinguistic Abilities—Revised

Reading and Spelling Tests

Diagnostic Spelling Potential Test

Test of Kindergarten/First Grade Readiness Skills (reading, spelling)

Gray Oral Reading Tests—3

Diagnostic Screening Test—Spelling

Diagnostic Screening Test—Reading

Test of Academic Achievement Skills

Diagnostic Achievement Battery

Test of Written Spelling—2 (grades 1-12)

Wide Range Achievement Test—3 Revised (reading, spelling, math)

Auditory Memory

Test of Memory and Learning (up to age 19)

Goldman-Fristoe-Woodcock Auditory Skills Test Battery

SCAN: A Screening Test for Auditory Processing Disorders, Following Directions subtest

Language-Structured Auditory Retention Span

Learning Efficiency Test—2

Auditory Discrimination

Wepman Auditory Discrimination Test

Goldman-Fristoe-Woodcock Auditory Skills Test Battery

Goldman-Fristoe-Woodcock Test of Auditory Discrimination, Quiet subtest

Auditory Figure-Ground (and/or auditory selective attention)

Goldman-Fristoe-Woodcock Auditory Skills Test Battery

Goldman-Fristoe-Woodcock Test of Auditory Discrimination

SCAN: A Screening Test for Auditory Processing Disorders (ages 13 to 30)

Auditory Cohesion (as defined in this book)

Detroit Test of Learning Aptitude—Adult

Test of Memory and Learning (5 to 19 years)

Wide Range Achievement Test—3 Revised

Auditory Attention

SCAN: A Screening Test for Auditory Processing Disorders (ages 13 to 30)

Quick Neurological Screening Test—Revised

Auditory Perception (as described in this book)

Caution: Some adults have not been taught reading via a phonic approach and may therefore experience difficulty with sound/symbol associations. This is different from an auditory perception problem in which sound and symbol correlations cannot be understood.

Diagnostic Spelling Potential Test

Additional insight in this area can be gained through the following tests:

Goldman-Fristoe-Woodcock Auditory Skills Test Battery, Reading subtest

Gray Oral Reading Tests—3 (ages 7 to 19)

Detroit Tests of Learning Aptitude—Adult

Minnesota Test for the Differential Diagnosis of Aphasia

Considerations When Writing the Diagnostic Evaluation Report

After testing and scoring are completed, the task of making sense of findings arises. What do the results mean in terms of the behaviors reported and observed? How do findings help to explain academic problems reported? What language-learning strategies may be recommended? What classroom and home modifications may be suggested? Is the child in the most appropriate classroom placement?

These and numerous other issues must be addressed. Without such applications, test results presented in isolation provide minimal help. Without effective communication of such findings and recommendations to the team members (parents, teachers, child, and others), the report remains a sterile document of little use. The basic focus becomes: How can problems be explained in terms of the results found, and how can these problems be best alleviated?

Each of the five main auditory processing skill areas must be examined. It is often appropriate also to comment on the relationships among skill areas. (For example, while auditory memory for sentences is adequate, the child may be unable to follow directions.) For many children, the "interpretation of directions" is different from mere recall of directed information in that it involves a higher-order manipulation of information, a response, and sometimes an ability to hold the direction in mind over time.

Therefore, the greatest challenges in the assessment process are to select appropriate assessment tools and to insightfully interpret and apply results. It is like a puzzle to be completed, and sometimes some of the pieces may be missing. The speech-language pathologist who has a working knowledge of classroom dynamics and curriculum issues is at an advantage.

Fundamental questions that relate to interpretation of results include but are not limited to:

1. How are spelling skills affected?

2. How are reading skills affected?

3. What classroom seating position is best for this child?

4. Are auditory figure-ground skills observed within normal limits (WNL)?

5. How may the classroom teacher modify his or her style of presenting material?

6. How are writing skills affected?

7. What presentation modifications can be made to facilitate the following of directions?

8. How do auditory discrimination, figure-ground, and/or auditory memory problems impact upon the following of directions?

9. How consistent are the problems displayed? What contexts cause the most problems? Why?

10. How can overall auditory attention be strengthened?

11. What instrumentation should be recommended, if any, and for what period of time and under what circumstances?

12. What are the long-term goals for the child? What can be started now to begin that process?

13. How is the child's self-esteem affected?

14. How has the child's CAP profile changed (if at all) over time?

Correlations of Specific Tests and Procedures with the Five Central Auditory Processing Skill Areas

The following outline represents the tests and informal procedures used in the various diagnostic evaluations in this book. These or other tests and procedures may be selected for this purpose. (See pages 39-41 for a more complete listing.) The listing below is representative and is not intended to be comprehensive. Interpretation of results is often complex and does not involve simply a direct correlation between test results and skill areas.

I. Auditory Memory:

   1. Test of Auditory Perceptual Skills

      Auditory number memory forward

      Auditory number memory reversed (possibly also applicable to skill area IV)

      Auditory sentence memory

      Auditory word memory

   2. Recall of nonsense syllable and word after 15 minutes (and 30 minutes)

   3. Recall of deferred direction after 15 minutes (and 30 minutes)

II. Auditory Discrimination:

   1. Goldman-Fristoe-Woodcock Test of Auditory Discrimination, Quiet subtest (involves a visual processing component)

   2. Test of Auditory Perceptual Skills

      Auditory word discrimination; auditory stimuli only

   3. Informal assessment of short-vowel identification, naming, and discrimination

III. Auditory Figure-Ground:

   1. Goldman-Fristoe-Woodcock Test of Auditory Discrimination, Noise subtest

   2. Informal observation (various noise stimuli and performance)

IV. Auditory Cohesion:

1. Test of Auditory Perceptual Skills

    Auditory interpretation of directions

    Auditory number memory reversed

    Auditory processing (thinking and reasoning)

2. Test of Auditory Reasoning and Processing Skills (when child is 5-14 years old)

V. Auditory Attention:

Informal procedures involving notation of auditory focus as functions of setting, content of materials, time, interest, and frustration levels, among other parameters

Vocabulary:

Peabody Picture Vocabulary Test—Revised (receptive vocabulary and possibly an indicator of overall language functioning)

Expressive One-Word Picture Vocabulary Test; also Upper Extension (expressive vocabulary)

Observations and comments relating to all five skill areas are drawn from the Case History Checklist (pages 81-82), the Child's Auditory Processing Skills Profile—Parent's Observations (pages 101-102) and the Child's Auditory Processing Skills Profile—Teacher's Observations (pages 117-118). Additional information often is drawn from the reports and observations of referral sources (for example, the referring pediatrician or psychologist), the school social worker, the nurse, and other team members. Other procedures involving spelling, syllabication, and reading decoding provide information about auditory processing skills from a broader perspective. These procedures are noted in the diagnostic evaluations in this chapter. See specific titles in this chapter for additional descriptions.

3

Diagnostic Specifics

Diagnostic Checklist

In assessing a child for possible central auditory processing disorder, the speech-language pathologist may mistakenly assume that processing is adequate based on evidence of one or more tests. For example, if one were to administer only the *Test of Auditory Perceptual Skills* (Gardner 1985) and fail to examine other skills such as auditory figure-ground abilities, it would be possible to come to a false-negative conclusion.

The checklist on page 46 may be used either before or after the diagnostic evaluation to make certain that the choice of assessment tools has reflected all the major areas of possible disorder. The choices selected in the various diagnostic profiles and summaries in this book are representative only.

Diagnostic Checklist

Child's Name:	Date:

Check or assess:

Auditory acuity skills	
Tympanometric status	
Developmental/medical/social/academic histories	
Child's perception of difficulties encountered, including likes and dislikes in school	
Oro-peripheral status	
Auditory memory for numbers	
Auditory memory for words	
Auditory memory for sentences	
Ability to interpret and follow immediate directions	
Ability to interpret and follow deferred directions	
Auditory discrimination (without a visual task component)	
Auditory discrimination (with a visual task component)	
Auditory attentional skills	
Auditory cohesion skills	
Auditory perception skills (as defined, including short- and long-vowel identification and discrimination)	
Spelling skills	
Reading decoding skills	
Oral reading skills (if applicable)	
Receptive vocabulary	
Expressive vocabulary	
Basic pragmatic skills	
Basic expressive and receptive language skills	
Parent's checklist	
Teacher's checklist	
Other areas of concern identified by teacher, parent, therapist	
Do your findings basically correlate (that is, make sense) with audiological results, parent/teacher checklists, and other speech-language testing?	
Have you accounted for any delimiting circumstances (for example, the child's attitude toward testing or status of health) that may have impacted on performance?	
Are findings from the informal, low-structured assessment procedures fairly consistent with those from high-structured procedures? If not, have you accounted for possible reasons?	

Deferred Auditory Memory Tasks

The following deferred recall tasks are grouped by degree of difficulty ranging from relatively simple tasks to more complex tasks. Each task can be documented in terms of time (How long after the initial command was the task acted upon?). This list may be used for several purposes. It may be used as part of the diagnostic evaluation to document how well the child is able to retain and act upon directions over time (5, 15, 30 minutes or longer). It also may be used to track progress in therapy by noting skill levels on particular dates. Finally, it may be used as part of the speech-language pathologist's progress summary or discharge report.

The list does not have to be used in its entirety. Also, the child must have some means of telling time if the therapist chooses not to cue the child at appropriate intervals. When a child cannot recall the task after a period of time, the possibility of poor auditory memory (as opposed to poor recall skills over time) should be examined. For a child who may not be able to recall information immediately, deferred recall is virtually impossible. Some children may have both immediate and deferred recall problems.

Deferred Auditory Memory Tasks

Name:	Date:

Place a check next to those items in which the child was cued in terms of time. In these cases, ask the child to "Clap your hands in five minutes," for example, and at the five-minute point, ask the child, "What did I ask you to do in five minutes?" This is considered less challenging than simply asking a child who is able to tell time, "After 5 minutes, clap your hands" and expecting the child to self-cue appropriately. A therapy program for deferred recall must start with short-term, cued recall of simple tasks and progress to long-term, self-cuing of complex tasks.

These tasks may be used as a basis for intervention materials devised by the clinician.

Verbal Recall Tasks:	5 minutes	15 minutes	30 minutes	Longer
1. Recall a one-syllable nonsense word.				
2. Recall a two-syllable nonsense word.				
3. Recall a three-syllable nonsense word.				
4. Recall a sentence of 6 words.				
5. Recall a sentence of 8 words.				
6. Recall a sentence of 10 words.				
7. Recall a riddle.				
8. Recall a phone number and address.				
9. Recall a nonsense sentence of 10 words.				
10. Recall a nonsense sentence of 12 words.				

Physical or Motor Tasks:				
1. Smile.				
2. Clap your hands.				
3. Touch your shoes.				
4. Blink your eyes three times.				
5. Draw a red circle.				
6. Draw a blue and green tree.				
7. Open and close the door twice.				
8. Open your mouth and touch your nose.				
9. Touch your left ear four times.				
10. Turn around three times while singing.				

Central Auditory Processing Disorder / Dorothy A. Kelly, D.A. / ISBN 0761631623

Graded Reading Word Lists

The following graded word lists are reprinted with permission from Scott, Foresman & Company. They are taken from the *Qualitative Reading Inventory* (1990) by Lauren Leslie and JoAnne Caldwell.

When assessing a child for possible central auditory processing disorder, lists may be used to observe the manner in which the child identifies words. Specifically, note strategies (or the lack of strategies) for word analysis. For example, does the child identify the correct number of syllables, accent appropriately, recognize morphological rules, distort vowels, and so on? The child with CAPD often has difficulty employing a phonics approach to reading. This procedure is most helpful when the child has not previously acquired the words via a sight-vocabulary approach (such as, memorized the visual configuration of the word rather than analyzing its components). Therefore, the task can be started at the present estimated grade level of performance, and progress to the more challenging level at which the child has not memorized or acquired a sight vocabulary. Since this is a relatively informal procedure, comments can be made on the diagnostic evaluation regarding performance at both the grade-level task and the postgrade-level task. Note whether a particular word was produced immediately (automatically) or "decoded."

These word lists range from the primer to junior high levels, with 20 words at each level. Limitations become apparent for children with CAPD whose performance levels may exceed junior-high levels. In children whose reading levels are higher than junior-high levels, the reading tool provided in this book will not be helpful. For example, an 11th-grade student may have a 10th-grade reading decoding level. Such a student probably would get 100% on a junior-high list of words. The one-year delay in reading level would not be identified.

Competency criteria involve the following factors:

1. At the postgrade level, is the child able to decode with a minimum of 70% to 85% accuracy? This score suggests a "working" competency for new words.

    If the child is unable to achieve 70% to 85% accuracy, it may be due to inadequate word analysis strategies.

2. At the performance grade level, is the child able to correctly identify 90% to 100% of the task words? This suggests a true competency for previously acquired words.

The issue of which approach to use when teaching reading skills is complex. While many children with CAPD appear to benefit most from a "see and say" or "sight" approach, in most cases elements of phonics approach should be incorporated into the child's reading program. Selection of these elements depends on the child's individual diagnostic profile. For example, the child's auditory discrimination skills are critical to success in learning from a phonics approach. If the child's auditory discrimination skills are deficient, a program for remediation is indicated which may ultimately allow the child to benefit from a phonics approach.

Although the "sight" approach provides some success, it is not the only option for children with CAPD. A particular child may be more receptive to aspects of a phonics approach (for example, syllabication skills) after therapy intervention. Phonics competency, in whatever form possible, will ultimately serve the child better than exclusive "sight" reading skills. This competency has positive effects on spelling, writing, reading comprehension, and learning foreign languages.

All children who demonstrate reading deficits should minimally be screened for possible auditory discrimination problems. A reading program that does not address the auditory discrimination problems may miss a fundamental basis for the child's failures.

Commercially produced oral reading inventories are also available. *Classroom Reading Inventory* (Silvaroli 1983) and *Qualitative Reading Inventory* (Leslie and Caldwell 1990), among others, offer graded paragraph selections which can be used to observe the child's oral reading skills. *How* a child reads aloud is very telling in terms of possible central auditory processing difficulties.

Have the child begin with a performance-level selection and progress to the next higher level. Observations may be made in terms of intonation (Does the pattern coordinate with grammatical markers and content?), vocal volume, rate, and word attack skills, among other areas. When problems are identified in these areas, therapy may focus on coordinating content or meaning of reading material with vocal expression that cues the meaning. The child may be taught how to identify signals or markers to meaning. (For example, the exclamation point usually indicates excitement and is orally coded with a louder voice and slightly elevated pitch level.)

A primary goal for the child with CAPD who exhibits reading difficulties is to increase association between the printed symbol and its auditory (and auditory perceptual) association. Such children often need qualitatively different intervention strategies than those used with other reading-impaired children. (Think *different* rather than *more.*) Where the more typical reading-impaired child may profit from repeated exposure to rules and examples, the child with CAPD often cannot. Chances are that the child has already been exposed to such rules and examples and they simply haven't been assimilated. Think *creatively,* perhaps employing multisensory techniques to reinforce associations.

Reading Word Lists

Primer	First	Second	Third	Fourh	Fifth	Sixth	Junior High
1. mother	1. friend	1. old	1. thread	1. weather	1. believed	1. sewed	1. tumultuous
2. went	2. run	2. toy	2. silk	2. settlers	2. protest	2. messenger	2. majestic
3. have	3. there	3. promise	3. tongue	3. precious	3. heaven	3. controlled	3. arduous
4. animal	4. then	4. trade	4. sharp	4. bend	4. managed	4. flee	4. navigated
5. what	5. find	5. pieces	5. rough	5. guarded	5. obey	5. championships	5. commissioned
6. saw	6. which	6. room	6. claws	6. pilot	6. convince	6. vowed	6. straits
7. some	7. school	7. built	7. believe	7. ocean	7. death	7. fortune	7. initiated
8. make	8. just	8. beach	8. crowded	8. conquer	8. sailor	8. memories	8. skirmish
9. was	9. bear	9. right	9. salmon	9. ruled	9. month	9. earthquake	9. reign
10. play	10. so	10. packed	10. hid	10. mounds	10. continue	10. abolish	10. bestowed
11. put	11. father	11. height	11. chief	11. signs	11. threatened	11. behavior	11. envious
12. every	12. rabbit	12. boards	12. whale	12. rescue	12. tales	12. volunteer	12. monarchy
13. children	13. great	13. measured	13. special	13. fought	13. laser	13. machines	13. sovereign
14. go	14. eat	14. branches	14. wool	14. bred	14. creature	14. organisms	14. laboriously
15. want	15. thought	15. though	15. removed	15. busy	15. heir	15. businesses	15. crucial
16. thing	16. tell	16. begins	16. lion	16. pond	16. wavelengths	16. shrinking	16. mantle
17. they	17. bread	17. push	17. wear	17. guide	17. statue	17. research	17. tsar
18. need	18. song	18. ends	18. lunch	18. escape	18. focuses	18. abdomen	18. dissolves
19. were	19. moved	19. front	19. curious	19. islands	19. tomb	19. environments	19. parliament
20. like	20. lake	20. morning	20. spin	20. fame	20. attend	20. slavery	20. reluctant

Analysis of Spelling Skills

The following word lists are broadly divided into two main categories: Lower-Level and Upper-Level words. These categories roughly correlate with primary school-age and secondary school-age (and beyond) students. Each broad category is further divided into lists which contain words that are "logical" (or generally spelled the way that they sound) and "less logical" (or generally not spelled the way that they sound). Each group of words contains 50 items. Administer two spelling tests from either the lower or upper levels, depending on the child's performance level in spelling. Ask the child to spell 20 words from both the "logical" and "less logical" lists to observe skills and strategies employed. For example:

> Does the child seem to rely solely upon visual memory when spelling?

> Does the child appear to use syllabication skills to analyze parts when spelling more challenging words?

> Does the child appear to confuse vowels when spelling?

> Does the child "talk himself through" a spelling task?

> Does the child seem to make logical mistakes?

> Does the child apply rules when spelling (for example, "i before e except after c")?

> Does the child evidence word attack or analysis skills when trying to spell a new word?

> Does the child apply words that are correctly spelled on classroom spelling tests to other writing tasks?

> Does the child appear to retain correct spellings once they have been acquired?

> Does the child seem to apply consistent and correct strategies to spelling tasks?

> Does the child seem to transport syllables (moving a syllable from one position in the word to another)?

> Does the child seem to omit or substitute phonemes or syllables?

> Does the child seem to speak the way he spells?

> Does the child like spelling tasks?

Information gathered through this informal procedure can provide another "piece of the puzzle." The child with central auditory processing disorder may have similar spelling and reading decoding patterns, and also may evidence poor sound-symbol associations, vowel and/or consonant discriminations, and syllabication skills that could be incorporated into a speech-language program. The program should be comprehensive and "whole language-like," recognizing that skills such as spelling, reading, speaking, and writing are often interrelated.

Lower-Level Word List

Logical Words	Less Logical Words	Logical Words	Less Logical Words
rug	ear	lip	year
see	eye	cup	true
big	rain	land	why
open	blue	butter	new
green	shoe	paper	walk
glass	touch	tap	speak
plant	hair	ten	was
seven	light	hold	dish
end	tie	and	phone
camp	island	sun	bear
send	friend	jump	high
pup	build	fun	buy
can	nation	hill	tooth
leg	tongue	mad	boat
find	mouth	just	they
hand	chair	feet	the
cap	juice	fast	meat
bend	two	bed	bread
post	one	me	sing
dress	very	hop	knee
carpet	much	sit	clean
red	our	mud	talk
rag	true	help	school
sister	easy	plus	should
milk	air	win	ready

Upper-Level Word List

This upper-level list contains words that are more challenging. The first group of 50 represent words that are spelled "logically" or generally as they sound. The second group of words are "less logical" and not spelled as they sound. These lists may be used in part for therapy purposes. Discussion may involve the logic or lack of logic for various spellings. Syllabication and prosodic cues may be stressed. Encourage the child to say each word aloud, listening to his or her own voice.

Logical Words	Less Logical Words	Logical Words	Less Logical Words
apparent	belief	operate	maneuver
strict	license	professor	absence
bulletin	conscious	suppress	augment
excellent	criticism	valuable	caught
considerably	deceive	record	thorough
interest	emphasize	summary	eighteen
practical	foreign	natural	neighborhood
history	straight	significant	machinery
remarkable	people	stapler	reception
illness	vengeance	diagnosis	language
slippery	fruit	format	breakdown
remember	spacious	rehabilitate	technical
lobster	Tuesday	bakery	someone
limited	feature	articulate	symbolism
fundamental	knowledge	public	measuring
happened	leisure	temporary	influential
across	physical	examine	issues
basis	ceiling	problematic	authors
category	occasion	assistant	impairments
dominant	fictitious	recommend	learning
permanent	theory	aggressive	therapeutic
hundred	maintenance	profile	scented
narrative	psychology	director	facilitation
attended	receive	compensate	achieve
ignorant	rhythm	clinical	resume

Sample Diagnostic Evaluation Reports

The following five sample diagnostic reports (pages 56-80) are representative of various types of profiles. The first report is one of a child who displayed some aspects of processing disorder on a very erratic basis. This profile suggested a possible underlying emotional component which complicated the diagnosis considerably. This child should be reexamined at a later point to see whether auditory processing symptoms continue after modifications of the listening and social environment are made. The other reports are representative of more typical cases of central auditory processing disorder.

The following tests were referred to in these diagnostic evaluation reports:

Dunn, L., and L. M. Dunn. 1981. *Peabody Picture Vocabulary Test—Revised*. Circle Pines, MN: American Guidance Service.

Gardner, M. F. 1979. *Expressive One-Word Picture Vocabulary Test*. Novato, CA: Academic Therapy Publications.

_____. 1985. *Test of Auditory Perceptual Skills*. San Francisco: Children's Hospital of San Francisco.

Goldman, R., M. Fristoe, and R. W. Woodcock. 1970. *Test of Auditory Discrimination*. Circle Pines, MN: American Guidance Service.

Child's Auditory Processing Skills Profile—Parent's Observations (see pages 101-102)

Child's Auditory Processing Skills Profile—Teacher's Observations (see pages 117-118)

Newcomer, Phyllis L., and Donald D. Hammill. 1982. *Test of Language Development—Primary*. Austin, TX: Pro-Ed.

Lower-Level Word List—Logical Words (see page 53)

Speech-Language Evaluation as per
Possible Central Auditory Processing Dysfunction

Date of Report: 5-29-95

Child's Name: Christopher Johnson

Date of Birth: 10-15-88

Date of Evaluation: 5-25-95

Background Information:

Christopher is an extremely bright 6-year, 7-month-old boy who currently resides with his mother. Although the full-term pregnancy was uncomplicated, delivery was by caesarian section due to fetal distress. The neonatal period was nonsignificant. Chris suffered from asthma which was treated with Proventyl elixir. He was hospitalized twice at ages 1½ and 2 years for rotoviral infections. During one of these events, Chris suffered a short-lived febrile seizure. As reported by the mother, Ms. Susan Lawrence, Chris suffered a concussion in September, 1993, after which his thinking became "fuzzy" and word-finding difficulties were noted. Apparently these symptoms have since been resolved. Chris has been taking Ritalin since October, 1994. Attention and behavior improvements have subsequently been noted at school. Ms. Lawrence indicated that he also experienced a few ear infections; however, pressure-equalizing tubes were not inserted. According to an audiological evaluation completed this week, hearing acuity falls within normal limits.

Chris currently attends kindergarten at a private school for the gifted. School problems have been reported in terms of behavior and attention. Similar difficulties were reported by Chris's mother, particularly in the area of following directions. Ms. Lawrence and Mr. Johnson (Chris's father) both noted that symptoms appear to worsen with pressure. Ms. Lawrence noted that when routines such as getting ready for school in the morning are allotted more time, tasks are completed with fewer problems. Chris reports that he likes school, particularly the subjects of math, science computers, and Spanish; however, he states that he doesn't like it "when the room becomes noisy." He states that he has difficulty concentrating at these times.

Chris has been tested in a number of settings with some inconsistent and conflicting findings. In terms of testing for central auditory processing, in April, 1994, Sandra Peters, Ph.D., found certain weaknesses in memory and strong auditory figure-ground and discrimination skills. In December, 1994, Anne O'Leary, M.S., speech-language pathologist, noted below-average auditory closure skills; other processing areas were identified as average to above average. Testing conducted in September, 1994, by behavioral psychologist Janet Simpson, Ph.D., yielded a diagnosis of Oppositional Defiant Disorder. A referral was made to this site by Dr. Simpson because of ongoing difficulties with following directions and other processing issues. Supplemental tutoring has been provided by Ms. Mary Brown, special education teacher, at Chris's school since April,

1995. The C.S.E. of Chris's school district has indicated a label of learning disabled for Chris at this point. Ms. Lawrence noted that the label was more exclusionary than diagnostic in that the district was uncertain as to any specific label. Ms. Lawrence is in the process of exploring educational options for next year (grade 1), since his present school has indicated that Chris cannot return in the fall because of the behavior problems.

A brief oro-peripheral examination noted a high, arched palate and malocclusion. A mild tongue thrust, sibilant distortions, and difficulty in producing the /r/ phoneme were noted. A mildly raspy vocal quality was also observed; Ms. Lawrence noted that this was not an ongoing quality. Speech was fluent, although slightly measured. Neither word-finding nor circumlocutions, as previously noted by Ms. Lawrence, were discovered.

Tests and Assessment Tools Administered:

Test of Auditory Perceptual Skills (assesses seven processing skills)

Auditory Number Memory:	L.A.	Percentile
Forward	>12 yrs.	99.9
Reversed	>12 yrs.	99.9
Auditory Sentence Memory	10 yrs. 8 mos.	98
Auditory Word Memory	>12 yrs.	99
Auditory Interpretation of Directions	9 yrs. 2 mos.	95
Auditory Word Discrimination	12 yrs.	84
Auditory Processing (thinking and reasoning)	>12 yrs.	99.6

Overall Auditory Quotient: 147

Overall Percentile Rank: 99+

Median Language Age: >12 yrs.

Goldman-Fristoe-Woodcock *Test of Auditory Discrimination*
(identifies possible auditory discrimination and figure-ground difficulties):

Quiet Subtest—Total errors: 1

Percentile rank: 73

Noise Subtest—Total errors: 6

Percentile rank: 96

Peabody Picture Vocabulary Test—Revised L (assesses receptive vocabulary skills):

Raw Score: 106

Age Equivalent: 9 yrs. 10 mos.

Standard Score Equivalent: 133

Percentile Rank: 99

Expressive One-Word Picture Vocabulary Test
(assesses expressive vocabulary skills):

Mental Age: 10 yrs. 3 mos.

Percentile Rank: 99+

Deviation I.Q.: 140

Reading Decoding Tool:

Primer level: 17 out of 20 correct; 85% accuracy

Child's Auditory Processing Skills Profile—Parent's Observations:

As completed by Ms. Lawrence, mild to moderate figure-ground problems, difficulties in following complicated directions, difficulties in maintaining overall attention, and problems with delayed recall/deferring action were identified.

Language Sample:

A brief language sample noted generally functional pragmatic and expressive language skills. Erratic eye contact was noted.

Informal Assessments:

A brief examination of deferred memory skills indicated normal functioning (at 5- and 10-minute intervals) in quiet environments.

Interpretation of Results:

Scores will be discussed in terms of five major categories of central auditory processing skills which impact on academic and social settings. These categories are: auditory figure-ground, auditory memory, auditory discrimination, auditory cohesion, and auditory attention.

Prior to testing, in an attempt to reduce pressure, Chris was assured that all efforts were acceptable. From that point, Chris appeared fairly relaxed, although he was quite concerned about the accuracy of his responses. Chris was able to maintain attention and effort for 1½ hours.

1. Auditory Figure-Ground Skills (the ability to screen out ambient or background noise distractions):

   As noted by the *Test of Auditory Discrimination* (and supported by testing completed by Dr. Peters), Chris does not appear to have a problem with ambient noise distractions. However, as discussed with Ms. Lawrence, although Chris "should not" be experiencing background noise difficulties, apparently Chris acts as if he did. This "secondary" figure-ground problem appears related to both the environment and stress. It is quite possible that in low stress environments, which are slow-paced and filled with praise and support, figure-ground symptoms will decrease.

2. Auditory Memory Skills (the ability to recall a variety of auditorily sequenced units):

   As indicated by the *Test of Auditory Perceptual Skills,* (number, sentence and word subtests) and the *Test of Language Development—Primary* (Sentence Imitation subtest), Chris does not evidence any type of auditory memory problem. In fact, skills were exceptional and consistent with levels of other processing skills. Any apparent inability to follow directions does not appear related to auditory memory deficits.

3. Auditory Discrimination Skills (the ability to note minor phonemic differences):

    As indicated by the "auditory discrimination" subtest of the *Test of Auditory Perceptual Skills,* Chris demonstrated excellent discrimination skills for auditorily produced word pairs. Additionally, scores noted by the *Test of Auditory Discrimination,* Quiet Subtest, suggest that even with a visual processing component, skills are above average.

4. Auditory Cohesion Skills (the ability to employ higher-order cognitive/processing skills in a meaningful manner):

    As evidenced by the "thinking and reasoning," "interpretation of directions," and "number memory reversed" subtests on the *Test of Auditory Perceptual Skills,* Chris appears to display very strong skills in this area. His ability to not only recall directions, but to apparently manipulate them meaningfully under ideal conditions, suggests that perhaps the difficulties noted at home and in school are not intrinsic.

5. Auditory Attention (the ability to maintain attention purposely even when interest may be limited; the ability to hold information and/or to defer action upon directions over time):

    Chris was able to attend to task items for 1½ hours, which suggests competent skills in overall attention under clinical conditions. Testing was prefaced with comments designed to diffuse stress and pressure. Chris was also successful in recalling a nonsense phrase after ½ hour. Although this is incomplete evidence, it does suggest an ability to retain information over time. Overall, Chris appears to display potentially normal skills in this area. However, there were minimal visual and auditory distractions within the test setting.

Summary of Results:

Perhaps most significant is the conspicuous absence of evidence regarding the auditory processing symptoms reported. "On paper," Chris presents an exceptionally strong and uniformly consistent auditory processing profile. Additionally, exceptionally strong expressive and receptive vocabulary skills are reflective of such high performance levels. However, Chris displays very specific behaviors which conflict with these findings. For example, although his reading decoding skills were appropriate for kindergarten, Chris's other skill areas far exceed this level of performance. Additionally, there was nothing noted by the testing (for example, poor auditory discrimination skills) that would account for this difference. This issue, however, is considered very minor. The other areas of confusion center around skills, such as auditory attention, following directions, and figure-ground, which are displayed erratically. Technically, Chris possesses above-average skills in these areas; yet in everyday experiences, he does not apply them functionally on a consistent basis. This profile suggests a possible emotional and/or attentional component, although other explanations also may be possible. This possible explanation should be further investigated by a psychologist.

Additionally, as evidenced by Ms. Lawrence's newfound success with the daily morning routine, many of Chris's "secondary symptoms" may be reduced by modifying expectations and manner of interaction. As discussed with Ms. Lawrence, although Chris is obviously a gifted child capable of exceptional academic success, perhaps he should be viewed first as a six-year-old child, with all the inconsistencies, fears, and immaturities expected at that age.

Recommendations:

Although academic challenge is certainly desirable for this bright child, at this point a comfortable and supportive educational environment seems far more important for Chris. Low-stress, structured academic and social environments filled with enjoyable peer interactions may yield fewer processing "symptoms." For these reasons, Chris is not a candidate for formal therapy at this site. However, it might be advantageous for parents and classroom staff to discuss specific modification techniques (for example, making requests calmly in "chunks," with little or low ambient noise distraction, while adding intonation and facial cues). It is also recommended that Chris be alerted to specific listening strategies so that when challenging tasks arise (for example, noisy environments), he can feel empowered to modify them as needed. With Chris taking an active, responsible role in recognizing and modifying his own listening environment, he may feel less pressured and frustrated and more in control. These measures should be viewed as transitional, to be discarded when application of skills to everyday tasks becomes more consistent. It is also recommended that Ms. Lawrence contact this clinician in three months to discuss progress. Additional recommendations may be made at that time.

Speech-Language Pathologist

Speech-Language Evaluation as per
Possible Central Auditory Processing Dysfunction

Date of Report: 11-20-95

Child's Name: John Smith

Date of Birth: 6-8-86

School: Kennedy Elementary School

Grade/Placement: 4th, special education

Date of Evaluation: 11-20-95

Referral Source/Reason for Evaluation: James Green, Ph.D., psychologist; to rule out central auditory processing dysfunction

Background Information:

John is a personable 9-year, 5-month-old boy who is the younger of two siblings within an intact family. He attended a special education preschool until age 5. He currently attends the fourth grade within a special education class and is labeled as learning disabled. Speech-language services had been provided five times weekly and more recently reduced to three times weekly with a new therapist. Services presently have been discontinued temporarily at the mother's request, due to a disagreement as to IEP goals and procedures.

Medical history is significant and includes a hospitalization for myringotomy and an attempted P.E. tube insertion in December, 1988. The latter procedure was aborted due to a septic condition; the tympanic membranes were "slashed," as reported by the mother. A tonsillectomy/adenoidectomy was completed in March, 1992. The mother also indicated that she experienced hypoglycemia during the last trimester of an otherwise normal pregnancy. Allergies were reported and include responses to cats, grass, and trees. John experienced two grand mal and two petit mal seizures, as reported by the mother. John also saw Jane Donahue, M.D., psychiatrist, at Shady Brook University Hospital.

Eyesight is reported as excellent. An audiological evaluation and tympanometric screening performed this week indicated within normal limits (WNL) of functioning bilaterally. John has not experienced an ear infection this year; however, a chronic history of otitis media has been ongoing and cyclical.

Mr. and Mrs. Smith brought John to this site at the recommendation of James Green, Ph.D., psychologist, who suspected central auditory processing involvement. The Smiths have indicated problems with complicated directions, background noise, and deferred directions, among other areas. Spelling, writing, and reading decoding skills are poor, while math skills appear stronger. John displays very low self-esteem (he identifies himself as "retarded") and indicates poor peer relationships.

Tests and Assessment Tools Administered:

Test of Auditory Perceptual Skills (assesses six processing skills):

	L.A.	Percentile
Auditory Number Memory		
Forward	>12 yrs.	95
Reversed	8 yrs. 4 mos.	37
Auditory Sentence Memory	7 yrs. 6 mos.	25
Auditory Word Memory	>12 yrs.	63
Auditory Interpretation of Directions	10 yrs. 8 mos.	75
Auditory Word Discrimination	>12 yrs.	91
Auditory Processing (thinking and reasoning)	11 yrs. 5 mos.	75

Overall Auditory Quotient: 11

Overall Percentile Rank: 77

Median Language Age: 11 yrs. 5 mos.

Goldman-Fristoe-Woodcock *Test of Auditory Discrimination* (identifies possible auditory discrimination and figure-ground difficulties):

Quiet Subtest—Total errors: 1

   Percentile rank: 63

   *1 pause

Noise Subtest—Total errors: 11

   Percentile rank: 30

Peabody Picture Vocabulary Test—Revised L (assesses receptive vocabulary skills):

Raw Score: 99

Age Equivalent: 8 yrs. 10 mos.

Standard Score Equivalent: 96

Percentile Rank: 39

Expressive One-Word Picture Vocabulary Test
(assesses expressive vocabulary skills):

Mental Age: 10 yrs. 11 mos.

Percentile Rank: 83

Deviation I.Q.: 114

Reading Decoding Tool:

First-grade level: 3 errors out of 20; 85% accuracy

---

*In excess of 5 pauses

Child's Auditory Processing Skills Profile—Parent's Observations:

Significant difficulties noted with background noises, excessive volume, visual distractions, complicated directions, deferred directions, and lengthy conversations.

Language Sample:

A brief language sample noted generally functional pragmatic skills. However, a tendency to avoid eye contact and go off conversational topic was noted. Expressive language skills appeared adequate, and rate of speech was noted as slow-normal.

A cursory oro-peripheral and articulation examination noted irregular dentition, a mildly high-arched palate, structures grossly adequate for speech purposes, and distortions of /r/ and /l/.

Additional Assessment Procedures:

Auditory memory (deferred) was informally assessed, using a nonsense word to be recalled after fifteen minutes. John was unable to complete this task on two occasions.

Auditory discrimination for short vowels and identification/recognition of short vowels was assessed. John displays competent skills in these tasks.

Spelling skills were informally observed. John does not appear to have functional syllabication or word attack strategies, and appears to use a sight-vocabulary approach to spelling and reading almost exclusively.

John had difficulty maintaining effort and focus throughout a 1¾-hour session and needed to be repeatedly brought back to task. However, his overall attitude was cooperative.

Interpretation of Results:

Scores will be discussed in terms of five major categories of central auditory processing skills which impact on academic and social settings. These categories are: auditory figure-ground, auditory memory, auditory discrimination, auditory cohesion, and auditory attention.

1. Auditory Figure-Ground Skills (the ability to screen out ambient or background noise distractions):

   As indicated by results of the Noise subtest of the Goldman-Fristoe-Woodcock *Test of Auditory Discrimination* (30th percentile), John displays a problem with background noise. This problem could exaggerate other existing problems. Additionally, because a child does not evidence problems with such areas as following directions or discrimination (for example, under more ideal circumstances such as those associated with this test session) does not necessarily mean that such problems could not surface with background noises. In fact, it is believed that John has such difficulty, as verified by anecdotal reports.

2. Auditory Memory Skills (the ability to recall a variety of auditorily sequenced units):

John appears to evidence strong auditory memory skills for numbers forward (l.a. >12 yrs. on the *Test of Auditory Perceptual Skills*) and words (l.a. >12 yrs. on the *Test of Auditory Perceptual Skills*). However, he demonstrates a problem with memory for sentences (l.a. 7 yrs. 6 mos. on the *Test of Auditory Perceptual Skills.*) This difficulty has obvious impact upon classroom performance, especially in the presence of background noise. John also appears to have problems carrying out deferred directions and recalling information over time.

3. Auditory Discrimination Skills (the ability to note minor phonemic differences):

As evidenced by the Quiet Subtest of the *Test of Auditory Discrimination* (63rd percentile), John has strong discrimination skills when a visual processing task is involved. Additionally, when only auditory discrimination of words is involved (*Test of Auditory Perceptual Skills* subtest), John continues to display strong skills (>12 yrs.). When short vowel contrasts are involved, skills again appear to be quite intact. This area appears to be a strength upon which individualized reading and spelling programs may rely.

4. Auditory Cohesion Skills (the ability to employ higher-order cognitive/ processing skills in a meaningful manner):

As evidenced by the "thinking and reasoning" subtest of the *Test of Auditory Perceptual Skills* (l.a. 11 yrs. 5 mos.), John displays strong skills in this higher-order processing area, suggesting significant fundamental cognitive skills. The auditory memory for numbers "reversed" subtest of the same test, which may be correlated with auditory cohesion, indicated below-average functioning (l.a. 8 yrs. 4 mos.). This area, however, is very frequently problematic for children (with and without processing disorders), and is not considered significant. Additionally, John displays above-average skills in the interpretation of directions (l.a. 10 yrs. 8 mos.), which also is suggestive of higher-order competencies. If John displays problems following directions or discriminating, it is probably due to setting (noisy environments) or attention rather than to deficient skills.

5. Auditory Attention (the ability to maintain attention purposely over an extended period of time):

John has a mild difficulty with overall auditory attention as functions of time, setting, and content of information. During testing, he had to be frequently called back to task and needed a break in order to continue. Considering his age, his testing behavior was not considered extraordinary, merely mildly problematic. With increased self-esteem and materials with which he could feel more successful, attention may increase to some extent.

Summary of Results:

John appears to display strong auditory processing skills in the areas of auditory memory for numbers and words. Auditory memory for sentences is significantly depressed. Strong skills were noted in auditory cohesion, discrimination, and interpretation of directions. Auditory figure-ground skills were found to be impaired. Such a deficiency probably impacts negatively upon other skills such as discrimination and memory. Deferred recall of auditory information was also found to be an area of difficulty. Expressive vocabulary skills are strong, and receptive vocabulary skills are mildly delayed. Overall, John displays considerable potential for growth.

Recommendations:

It is very important that John's auditory figure-ground difficulties be addressed. An auditory trainer may be used in limited contexts if acceptable to John. However, use of this device should be transitional and temporary. Therapy should focus on building figure-ground skills first within the therapy environment, and then within the classroom. Auditory memory for sentences should also be improved, as well as deferred recall and following directions in noise. Reading and spelling approaches should be modified to reflect a combination of phonics and sight approaches. Auditory cues, such as intonation and rate markers, should be identified and explained for John. Self-esteem issues also impact heavily upon performance and effort.

Therapy is recommended for two individual periods weekly to address the areas specified.

_____

Speech-Language Pathologist

Speech-Language Evaluation as per
Possible Central Auditory Processing Dysfunction

Date: December 18, 1995

Child's Name: Russell Burns

Date of Birth: July 5, 1984

School: West Side Junior High

Grade/Placement: 6th grade/regular

Date of Evaluation: December 18, 1995

Referral Source/Reason for Evaluation: Mary Benson, Ph.D., psychologist

Background Information:

Russell is a quiet, pleasant, 11-year, 5-month-old, left-handed boy who resides with his parents and one older brother. He attends the sixth grade in the West Side Junior High School. He likes math, social studies, reading, English, and gym, and dislikes science. He is currently maintaining a B average; however, some teachers have reported difficulties in following directions and focusing. Mrs. Ellen Burns, mother, reported that Russell frequently asks, "What?" and appears to "mishear" directions and information. Russell stated that noisy settings seem to make listening more difficult for him. Mrs. Burns also noted that Russell appears to have difficulties understanding abstract materials and completing assignments, and he seems to lack appropriate logic at times. She also noted that he displayed mixed laterality until kindergarten and beyond, although she considers him athletic and coordinated. Russell's parents had him evaluated by Mary Benson, Ph.D., to clarify these concerns. Dr. Benson noted during the course of testing that visual processing tasks appeared problematic, especially when coupled with an auditory component. Intelligence testing yielded an overall score of 86, which grossly agreed with testing completed by the school district. Russell's mother stated that he has always had a problem in taking standardized tests and that the school personnel felt the low scores did not represent his true potentials. Mrs. Burns stated that math and vocabulary scores are typically deficient on such tests. She also noted that Russell's self-esteem and peer relationships are good. Medical history is largely nonsignificant. However, Russell suffers from mild asthma and sinus difficulties. In infancy, he had one ear infection, accompanied by pain and high fever. Treatment was limited to the use of antibiotics and ear drops. An oro-peripheral examination was nonsignificant, indicating structures adequate for speech purposes. An audiological evaluation with tympanometry completed this week indicated within normal limits of functioning.

Tests and Assessment Tools Administered:

Test of Auditory Perceptual Skills (assesses six processing skills):

Auditory Number Memory	L.A.	Percentile
Forward	>12 yrs.	63
Reversed	10 yrs. 4 mos.	25
Auditory Sentence Memory	8 yrs. 9 mos.	16
Auditory Word Memory	6 yrs. 11 mos.	9
Auditory Interpretation of Directions	9 yrs. 2 mos.	25
Auditory Word Discrimination	11 yrs. 6 mos.	50
Auditory Processing (thinking and reasoning)	10 yrs. 6 mos.	25

Overall Auditory Quotient: 88

Overall Percentile Rank: 21

Median Language Age: 10 yrs. 4 mos.

Goldman-Fristoe-Woodcock *Test of Auditory Discrimination*
(identifies possible auditory discrimination and figure-ground difficulties):

Quiet Subtest—Total errors: 4

Percentile rank: 5

Noise Subtest—Total errors: 8

Percentile rank: 49

Peabody Picture Vocabulary Test—Revised L (assesses receptive vocabulary skills):

Raw Score: 90

Age Equivalent: 7 yrs. 10 mos.

Standard Score Equivalent: 71

Percentile Rank: 3

Expressive One-Word Picture Vocabulary Test
(assesses expressive vocabulary skills):

Mental Age: 11 yrs. 8 mos.

Percentile Rank: 58

Deviation I.Q.: 103

Reading Decoding Tool:

19/20 items correctly identified at the sixth-grade level

Child's Auditory Processing Skills Profile—Parent's Observations:

As indicated by the mother, Russell demonstrates severe difficulties with delayed recall of directions and understanding abstract information. He exhibits moderate difficulties with overall auditory attention and auditory processing with a visual task component.

Behaviors in Children with Central Auditory Processing Disorders— A Checklist for the Classroom Teacher:

Problems were noted in following directions, overall attention, and delayed recall, among other areas.

Language Sample:

Expressive language skills appear generally functional for conversation purposes. A tendency to avoid eye contact was noted. Mild sibilant and /r/ distortions were noted.

Additional Assessment Procedures:

Several informal procedures were completed, including a task requiring delayed recall (after 15 minutes) of a nonsense word. Russell was able to recall a nearly exact rendition of the word. He was also asked to describe the process of completing a hypothetical school assignment as well as one other complicated procedure. These procedures were designed to examine possible executive dysfunction behaviors, since this was an issue raised by parents and teachers. Russell was able to adequately break down the task into manageable steps. This possible problem, however, should be examined fully.

Russell was also asked to identify the short-vowel sounds and discriminate among them. He displayed difficulty in identifying the phonemes as produced by the clinician. Mrs. Burns felt that this was because he had not identified such phonemes for several years and had simply forgotten the sound/symbol associations. Russell was successful in identifying the number of syllables in polysyllabic words. He was then asked to spell various words, some of which were not spelled as they sounded and some of which were new to him. Russell appears to have a working ability to complete such tasks successfully. These latter procedures, although informal, suggest functional abilities in auditory perception (sound/symbol associations).

Interpretation of Results:

Scores will be discussed in terms of five major categories of central auditory processing skills which impact on academic and social settings. These categories are: auditory figure-ground, auditory memory, auditory discrimination, auditory cohesion, and auditory attention.

1. Auditory Figure-Ground Skills (the ability to screen out ambient or background noise distractions):

   As evidenced by results on the Noise Subtest of the Goldman-Fristoe-Woodcock *Test of Auditory Discrimination* (49th percentile), Russell appears to have functional skills in this area. If he displays problems in following directions, it is more likely due to deficient memory and/or interpretation skills rather than auditory figure-ground difficulties (or auditory discrimination problems as explained below). The problem presented by visual distractions should be examined.

2. Auditory Memory Skills (the ability to recall a variety of auditorily sequenced units):

As indicated by various subtests of the *Test of Auditory Perceptual Skills,* including the auditory number memory reversed subtests (l.a. 10 yrs. 4 mos.), interpretation of directions subtest (l.a. 9 yrs. 2 mos.), word memory subtest (l.a. 6 yrs. 11 mos.), and sentence memory subtest (l.a. 8 yrs. 9 mos.), Russell displays significant auditory memory difficulties. The first two subtests identified above also may be correlated with higher-order auditory cohesion skills.

3. Auditory Discrimination Skills (the ability to note minor phonemic differences):

As indicated by the auditory discrimination subtest of the *Test of Auditory Perceptual Skills,* Russell displays average skills in this area (l.a. 11 yrs. 6 mos.). When the task of discrimination involves a visual component, as in the *Test of Auditory Discrimination* (Quiet Subtest), skills dissipate significantly (5th percentile). This discrepancy suggests basically good auditory discrimination skills and possible auditory/ visual processing problems.

4. Auditory Cohesion Skills (the ability to employ higher-order cognitive/ processing skills in a meaningful manner):

As indicated by the "thinking and reasoning" subtest of the *Test of Auditory Perceptual Skills* (l.a. 10 yrs. 6 mos.), as well as comments made above in #1, Russell exhibits difficulties in this skill area. These findings support observations made by Russell's mother on the parent's checklist.

5. Auditory Attention (the ability to maintain attention purposely over an extended period of time):

Russell was able to maintain attention for approximately 1½ hours during the test session. This setting was relatively distraction-free, and he was repeatedly encouraged to maintain eye contact. Russell's auditory attention decreases in settings which contain visual distractions and tasks requiring strong auditory memory and/or cohesion skills.

Summary of Results:

Russell scored more poorly on the *Peabody Picture Vocabulary Test—Revised L,* which involves auditory/visual processing of multipicture tasks, than he did on the *Expressive One-Word Picture Vocabulary Test.* He also scored more poorly on the Quiet Subtest of the *Test of Auditory Discrimination* (which had a similar auditory/visual component) than on the auditory discrimination subtest of the *Test of Auditory Perceptual Skills.* These findings appear consistent with observations made by Dr. Benson, who suggested possible difficulties in coordinating simultaneous auditory and visual stimuli.

Russell displays significant problems with auditory memory for sentences, numbers—reversed, word memory, and the ability to interpret directions. Number memory for numbers—forward appears quite strong. Auditory cohesion skills appear delayed by approximately one year. Such findings are consistent with observations made by the parents regarding poor auditory logic and abstractions. No evidence of auditory latency (slowed processing) was noted. This observation, as reported by the mother, is more likely related to that fact that Russell is a sensitive child who "weighs" his responses carefully before responding. Receptive vocabulary skills appear delayed; however, this weak showing may be related to deficient auditory/visual processing more than to deficient vocabulary. This possibility may also confirm Mrs. Burns's observation that Russell is a poor test-taker and his teacher's belief that test scores did not represent his true abilities. Strong skills were noted in expressive vocabulary.

Recommendations:

Russell should develop the habit of establishing consistent eye contact with speakers in order to exploit natural speech-reading cues. He should be seated toward the front of the classroom with his back to the windows in order to limit visual distractions and facilitate natural speech-reading. Parents and teachers should present extended directions with slightly exaggerated intonation, natural expressive gestures, and facial expressions. Presentations should be made with a slightly elevated vocal volume and slightly slowed rate.

Russell is a candidate for therapy (three times weekly if within the school setting) which addresses these concerns. Memory and interpretation of directions should become the first priorities. Auditory and visual difficulties should be examined in greater depth with the possibility of intervention in this area. Auditory cohesion and vocabulary problems should be addressed subsequently. A psychologist may be consulted regarding possible concerns about self-esteem.

Speech-Language Pathologist

Speech-Language Evaluation as per
Possible Central Auditory Processing Dysfunction

Date: November 29, 1995

Child's Name: Daniel Cameron

Date of Birth: 4-05-85

School: Branchbrook Elementary School

Grade/Placement: 5th grade/regular

Date of Evaluation: 11-29-95

Background Information:

Daniel is a pleasant 10-year, 7-month-old boy who resides with his mother, father, and 14-year-old sister. He currently attends the fifth grade at Branchbrook Elementary School. Mrs. Jane Cameron, mother, reported that although Daniel's grades are basically good, his teacher, Mrs. Ames, reported problems with shyness, attention, following directions, organization, and completing tasks. Reportedly, Daniel likes science, computers, and electronics; he dislikes math and reading. Spelling and decoding skills, according to his mother, are adequate, although handwriting is poor. Daniel indicated that he disliked school in general, but enjoyed gym and recess. Mrs. Cameron corroborated his apparent lack of interest in school, but reported that he has several good friends this year in his class.

Mrs. Cameron indicated that similar problems also are noted at home. However, she stated that he "becomes a different person" when the task is related to an area of interest to him. For example, he "absorbs and retains computer commands easily and rapidly." Mrs. Cameron also indicated that Daniel attended a speech-language program in preschool, but since entrance into his present school has not received any special services other than resource room for math. She also stated that Daniel's first grade teacher had felt that he was perhaps "autistic or deaf." This was based on observations of shyness and inattentiveness. Other behaviors noted by Mrs. Cameron include difficulties with background noises, "mishearing" content of directions and conversations, and difficulties in carrying out deferred directions. She also felt that Daniel's self-esteem was poor. Reportedly, the elder sibling does well academically in school and displays no such behaviors.

Mr. and Mrs. Cameron sought psychological services when Daniel was in first grade. Services were not continuous since that time; however, recently a diagnosis of attention deficit disorder (without hyperactivity) was made. A referral was made to this site to further clarify those aspects of inattention related to auditory processing.

Daniel's medical history includes six ear infections from birth to age 18 months. Treatment was limited to the use of antibiotics. He is allergic to the Cephalosporin group of antibiotics (Keflex, etc.). Mrs. Cameron reported a normal pregnancy and delivery. She also reported that Daniel had sustained a dog bite to the face, for which he received medical treatment. Daniel's hearing and tympanometric status were evaluated this week and found to be normal.

Tests and Assessment Tools Administered:

Test of Auditory Perceptual Skills (assesses six processing skills):

Auditory Number Memory	L.A.	Percentile
Forward	11 yrs. 7 mos.	50
Reversed	6 yrs. 2 mos.	5
Auditory Sentence Memory	8 yrs. 9 mos.	25
Auditory Word Memory	6 yrs. 11 mos.	16
Auditory Interpretation of Directions	9 yrs. 2 mos.	25
Auditory Word Discrimination	>12 yrs.	84
Auditory Processing (thinking and reasoning)	>12 yrs.	75

Overall Auditory Quotient: 93

Overall Percentile Rank: 32

Median Language Age: 9 yrs. 2 mos.

Test of Auditory Discrimination
(identifies possible auditory discrimination and figure-ground difficulties):

Quiet Subtest—Total errors: 1

Percentile rank: 58th

*0 pauses

Noise Subtest—Total errors: 9

Percentile rank: 38th

Peabody Picture Vocabulary Test—Revised L (assesses receptive vocabulary skills):

Raw Score: 113

Age Equivalent: 10 yrs. 10 mos.

Standard Score Equivalent: 102

Percentile Rank: 55

Expressive One-Word Picture Vocabulary Test
(assesses expressive vocabulary skills):

Mental Age: 12 yrs. 3 mos.

Percentile Rank: 79

Deviation I.Q.: 112

Reading Decoding Tool:

4 out of 20 errors at the 4th grade level: 80% accuracy

---

*5 pauses

Child's Auditory Processing Skills Profile—Parent's Observations:

Difficulties noted in areas of auditory memory, interpretation of directions, auditory figure-ground, delayed recall of information, and auditory attention, among other areas.

Behaviors in Children with Central Auditory Processing Disorders—A Checklist for the Classroom Teacher:

Completed and indicated difficulties with following directions, organization, listening comprehension, and attention, among other areas.

Language Sample:

A brief language sampling indicated adequate expressive language skills and basically functional conversation skills, with the exception of poor eye contact and apparent shyness. A cursory oroperipheral examination noted structures grossly adequate for speech purposes. Mild sibilant distortions were noted.

Additional Assessment Procedures:

Informal procedures included the recall of a nonsense word after 15 minutes. Daniel was unsuccessful in this task twice. He was also asked to describe the processes of getting ready for school in the morning and making a peanut butter and jelly sandwich. He was accurate in these tasks. Additionally, he was able to identify the short vowels when named, discriminate among them, and name them. He also was asked to spell both logically and illogically constructed words at and below his estimated grade level. He was able to correctly spell approximately 50% of the words, with equal difficulty with both groups.

Interpretation of Results:

Scores will be discussed in terms of five major categories of central auditory processing skills which impact on academic and social settings. These categories are: auditory figure-ground, auditory memory, auditory discrimination, auditory cohesion, and auditory attention.

1. Auditory Figure-Ground Skills (the ability to screen out ambient or background noise distractions):

   As indicated by the *Test of Auditory Discrimination* (Noise Subtest; 38th percentile) as well as anecdotal reports from both the mother and the child himself, Daniel has a significant problem in noisy settings. When this problem is coupled with auditory memory and interpretation of directions difficulties, classroom functioning is very frustrating. Such a complex problem may easily impact upon auditory attention, distractibility, and attitude. It was necessary to stop the *Test of Auditory Discrimination* (Noise Subtest) five times due to Daniel's inability to complete the task. He appeared very stressed by this procedure. He did not need to pause at all for the auditory discrimination subtest on the same test.

2. Auditory Memory Skills (the ability to recall a variety of auditorily sequenced units): As indicated by reports from the classroom teacher, parent, and results of the *Test of Auditory Perceptual Skills,* Daniel displays significant auditory memory problems. On the *Test of Auditory Perceptual Skills,* he demonstrates an auditory sentence memory of 8 yrs. 9 mos., an auditory

word memory of 6 yrs. 11 mos., and an auditory memory for numbers reversed of 6 yrs. 2 mos. (See #4 below for further comment on this area.) These deficits may negatively impact upon tasks related to lectures, directions, and conversations, among numerous other areas. Such deficits tend to become worsened in noisy settings.

3. Auditory Discrimination Skills (the ability to note minor phonemic differences):

As indicated by the auditory word discrimination subtest of the *Test of Auditory Perceptual Skills* (l.a. >12 yrs.), Daniel displays strong skills when the task is exclusively auditorily based. He demonstrates relatively strong skills when a visual task is also involved, as evidenced by results on the *Test of Auditory Discrimination* (Quiet Subtest; 58th percentile). Programs that involve a multisensory basis would be beneficial to Daniel, especially since he clearly enjoys mechanically and physically oriented activities. Such an approach may encourage longer attention spans.

4. Auditory Cohesion Skills (the ability to employ higher-order cognitive/ processing skills in a meaningful manner):

As indicated by the "thinking and reasoning" subtest of the *Test of Auditory Perceptual Skills* (l.a. >12 yrs.), Daniel displays strong skills in this higher-order area. However, his ability to interpret directions (l.a. 9 yrs. 2 mos.) and auditory number memory reversed (l.a. 6 yrs. 2 mos.) are deficient. The former score may partially reflect Daniel's interest in science, competent vocabulary skills, and solid foundation of basic information skills.

5. Auditory Attention (the ability to maintain attention purposely over an extended period of time):

Daniel's attention appeared generally adequate for the 1½-hour test session. He needed to be prompted to return to task occasionally, and he needed a brief break. However, overall attention did not seem significantly impaired. The test environment was quiet, one-to-one, and supportive of efforts.

Summary of Results:

Daniel displays competent expressive and receptive vocabulary skills. Some aspects of central auditory processing are strong, including number memory forward, auditory discrimination, and "thinking and reasoning" skills. However, other processing skills are problematic, including sentence and word memories, interpretation of directions, delayed recall, and auditory figure-ground skills. Reading decoding and spelling skills appear mildly delayed and probably related to weak word attack strategies. Prognosis for remediation is considered good.

Recommendations (in addition to those above):

Therapy is recommended for two individual periods per week. An auditory trainer, to be used selectively as a transitional device until auditory figure-ground skills are strengthened, is an option, contingent upon Daniel's tolerance within the classroom. Preferential seating is recommended, and small-group interactions are encouraged as much as possible. Techniques such as intonation cuing, which facilitate recall, should be used by the teacher and parents. Daniel should establish eye contact with speakers to activate natural speech-reading cues. Organizational strategies are recommended, such as making chore lists, using an assignment pad, and maintaining a neat desk.

Speech-Language Pathologist

Speech-Language Evaluation as per
Possible Central Auditory Processing Dysfunction

Date of Report: May 25, 1995

Child's Name: Andrew Gordon

Date of Birth: 7-2-87

School: Frances Thomas Elementary School

Grade: 2nd

Date of Evaluation: May 23, 1995

Background Information:

Andrew is a personable 7-year, 10-month-old boy who resides with both parents and two siblings. He currently attends the Frances Thomas Elementary School, where he is a second grader. He will be retained next year. Since first grade, he has received private tutoring for academic reinforcement, primarily reading. Andrew experiences reading decoding/comprehension problems, and in the past has had difficulty with sound associations and discrimination, especially short vowels. Additional problems with spelling and writing are noted. Andrew indicated that he dislikes reading but enjoys math computation (not verbal math problems).

Mrs. Elizabeth Gordon, mother, reported a severe history of middle-ear pathology which began at two months of age and included the use of various antibiotics, an adenoidectomy/tonsillectomy, and two myringotomies. Mrs. Gordon was told that Andrew "always had fluid in his ears." Andrew is allergic to penicillin. Mrs. Gordon suspects other allergies. A history of asthma was reported. Vision has been tested and found to be normal. Hearing was evaluated on 5-20-95 and also found to be normal. Mrs. Gordon has indicated that a younger male sibling appears to evidence processing symptoms similar to Andrew's.

Andrew was examined at Milford Eye, Ear, and Throat Hospital on 2-13-95 and found to exhibit good speech recognition even for distorted speech, but significantly depressed skills in the presence of competing signals. A personal FM system for use in the classroom, preferential seating, and auditory training were recommended. Andrew was also examined by a speech-language pathologist at the family's group medical center. No significant problems were identified at the latter site, while significant auditory figure-ground difficulties were discovered at the former site. John Conti, audiologist, Port Smith Hearing and Speech Center, fitted Andrew with a Telex Personal Listening System on 4-11-95. The classroom teacher has indicated improvements in Andrew's ability to attend and follow directions.

Mrs. Gordon reported that at home Andrew has problems following directions, interpreting complex higher-order auditory information, retaining information and directions over time, and processing in the presence of ambient noise (or visual distractions), among other difficulties. He is very uncomfortable with loud auditory stimuli. Small-group and one-to-one interactions are preferred. Skills degenerate further when Andrew is tired. Mrs. Gordon noted that his self-esteem is low and social relationships are erratic.

A brief oroperipheral examination noted a mildly reversed swallow pattern and structures grossly adequate for speech purposes. A slightly arched palate was noted. Mrs. Gordon reported that Andrew had been a thumbsucker.

Mrs. Gordon brought Andrew to this site for a language-based, central auditory processing evaluation in order to further confirm and clarify these problems and to identify a specific program for remediation, if appropriate.

Overall auditory attention and effort during the test period of 1½ hours were considered adequate.

Tests and Assessment Tools Administered:

Test of Auditory Perceptual Skills (assesses six processing skills):

Auditory Number Memory	L.A.	Percentile
Forward	8 yrs. 3 mos.	50
Reversed	<4 yrs.	9
Auditory Sentence Memory	7 yrs. 6 mos.	63
Auditory Word Memory	4 yrs. 5 mos.	25
Auditory Interpretation of Directions	9 yrs. 2 mos.	84
Auditory Word Discrimination	>12 yrs.	91
Auditory Processing (thinking and reasoning)	5 yrs. 8 mos.	5

Overall Auditory Quotient: 97

Overall Percentile Rank: 42

Median Language Age: 7 yrs. 6 mos.

Goldman-Fristoe-Woodcock *Test of Auditory Discrimination*
(identifies possible auditory discrimination with a visual task component and figure-ground difficulties):

Quiet Subtest—Total errors: 2

Percentile rank: 42

Noise Subtest—Total errors: 13

Percentile rank: 19

Peabody Picture Vocabulary Test—Revised L (assesses receptive vocabulary skills):

Raw Score: 82

Age Equivalent: 7 yrs. 1 mo.

Standard Score Equivalent: 90

Percentile Rank: 25

Note: Children with CAPD sometimes have lower-than-expected receptive language scores in relation to expressive vocabulary scores.

Expressive One-Word Picture Vocabulary Test
(assesses expressive vocabulary skills):

> Mental Age: 7 yrs. 2 mos.
>
> Percentile Rank: 30
>
> Deviation I.Q.: 92
>
> Graded Reading Decoding Tool:
>
> 13 out of 20 errors at the second-grade level: 35% accuracy

Child's Auditory Processing Skills Profile—Parent's Observations:

Mother reported moderate to severe problems with following directions, retaining information over time, interpreting abstract information, and noise intolerances, among other observations. Skills improve when the child attends to the speaker's face.

Andrew tends to be forgetful and disorganized (characteristics common to children with CAPD).

Behaviors in Children with Central Auditory Processing Disorders— A Checklist for the Classroom Teacher:

Teacher reports difficulties with attention, following directions in noise, organization, writing from dictation, spelling, and reading, among other areas.

Language Sample:

A brief language sample noted a mild frontal lisp, sibilant distortions, generally adequate expressive language, and functional pragmatic skills.

Additional Assessment Procedures:

Andrew was successful 50% of the time in deferred auditory memory tasks which required him to recall a nonsense word after five minutes.

Andrew was able to identify all the short vowels and discriminate among them with 100% accuracy.

Andrew evidenced great difficulty when asked to spell various selections from the Lower-Level Word List—Logical Words, suggesting possible correlative reading encoding difficulties and auditory perception limitations. A pattern of types of errors could not be determined, because Andrew typically responded, "I have no idea," rather than attempt to encode. Possible patterns should be explored further, because such patterns often provide additional information about a child's auditory processing deficits. Reading and spelling programs that are sensitive to processing deficits tend to be more successful for children with CAPD.

Interpretation of Results:

Scores will be discussed in terms of five major categories of central auditory processing skills which impact on academic and social settings. These categories are: auditory figure-ground, auditory memory, auditory discrimination, auditory cohesion, and auditory attention.

1. Auditory Figure-Ground Skills (the ability to screen out ambient or background noise distractions):

   As evidenced by results on the Goldman-Fristoe-Woodcock *Test of Auditory Discrimination* (Noise Subtest; 19th percentile), Andrew demonstrates a significant problem with ambient noise. This finding is supported by test results at Milford Eye, Ear, and Throat Hospital as well as the classroom teacher's and the mother's anecdotal observations. Although the ability to interpret immediate directions (as indicated on the *Test of Auditory Perceptual Skills*) may be intact, such skills decrease markedly in noise. Such difficulties are further complicated by memory problems as described below. In effort, poor memory skills become even further impaired in ambient noise. The number—reversed memory task has implications for the Auditory Cohesion category noted below. The child is required not only to recall a sequence of numbers but to manipulate them in the mind in order to produce the sequence in reverse.

2. Auditory Memory Skills (the ability to recall a variety of auditorily sequenced units):

   As evidenced by the auditory word subtest of the *Test of Auditory Perceptual Skills,* Andrew appears to exhibit poor memory for isolated words (4 yrs. 5 mos.) and numbers reversed (<4 yrs.), while demonstrating stronger skills for sentences (7 yrs. 6 mos.) and numbers forward (8 yrs. 3 mos.). The use of syntactical context cues appear to help him recall sentence structures. Therapy may exploit these cues (in addition to exaggerated intonation and rhythm cues) to expand memory skills. Because a child evidences intact memory for sentences does not necessarily indicate that he can carry out directions, immediate or delayed.

3. Auditory Discrimination Skills (the ability to note minor phonemic differences):

   As evidenced by the Quiet Subtest on the *Test of Auditory Perceptual Skills* (l.a. >12 yrs.), Andrew demonstrates very strong skills when only auditory contrasts are provided. Skills dissipate to a degree when a visual task is required, as on the Goldman-Fristoe-Woodcock *Test of Auditory Discrimination* (42nd percentile). When required to coordinate both visual and auditory tasks, skills decrease. This is possibly related to Andrew's reading and spelling difficulties. Reading programs should reflect recognition of this contrast by having Andrew watch the speaker's face, isolating modes as needed; and by augmenting syllabication and intonation cues.

4. Auditory Cohesion Skills (the ability to employ higher-order cognitive/processing skills in a meaningful manner):

   As evidenced by the thinking and reasoning (l.a. 5 yrs. 8 mos.) and the numbers—reversed memory (l.a. <4 yrs.) subtests on the *Test of Auditory Perceptual Skills,* Andrew appears to display significant deficits in this area. Supporting this observation, his mother reported that he had severe difficulties with abstract and logic-based information.

Children with CAPD who lack more fundamental, lower-order processing skills, such as aspects of auditory memory, typically score poorly in this area. Therapy may involve the building of lower-order skills first, so that higher-order skills may be established more naturally.

5. Auditory Attention (the ability to maintain attention purposely over an extended period of time):

Andrew's overall auditory attention within the quiet confines of the test environment appeared adequate. Attention decreases in noise and over time when tasks become difficult.

Summary of Results:

Andrew displays significant deficits in auditory word and numbers reversed memories, auditory cohesion, and auditory figure-ground skills. He is able to follow immediate directions in quiet; however, deferred recall of information is poor. Overall attention in one-to-one settings appears adequate. Both receptive and expressive vocabulary deficits are noted.

Recommendations (in addition to those above):

1. Use of the personal auditory trainer is supported as a transition tool only until auditory figure-ground skills may be developed in therapy. It should be used only within the classroom and for specific purposes. Tolerance to background noise should be gradually increased in therapy through exposure to three or four categories of noise while increasingly complicated tasks are executed.

2. Andrew is a candidate for therapy. Therapy should include organizational strategies, syllabication techniques, recall tools of reauditorization and subvocalization, and parent/teacher involvement.

3. Andrew should be actively involved in identifying difficult listening environments and modifying them to the extent possible. Organizational strategies should be applied both at home and at school. He should routinely apply natural speech-reading techniques.

4. Preferential seating and small-group and one-to-one interactions are recommended in the classroom.

5. Continued medical monitoring of the middle-ear status and impact on hearing should continue.

_____

Speech-Language Pathologist

Case History Checklist

Child's Name:	Date:

The following questions may be used to supplement other case history information.

1. Did (or does) the child have a history of ear infections?

   If yes, when were the infections?

   How many were there?

   How were they treated?

   What were the typical symptoms?

   How long did a typical ear infection last?

   Did the child seem to speak less frequently during an infection period?

   How long after medication began did the symptoms continue during any typical infection?

   Did you notice any decrease in hearing ability during a typical infection?

   If yes, was the child able to identify that hearing was poorer?

   Was the child's hearing tested during the time of infections?

   If yes, what were the results?

2. Does the child have any allergies?

   If yes, please specify.

(continued)

Central Auditory Processing Disorder / Dorothy A. Kelly, D.A. / ISBN 0761631623

3. Does the child tolerate noisy settings well?

   If no, please specify.

4. Does the child seem to frequently "mishear" directions or the content of conversations?

   If yes, please specify.

5. Does the child have difficulty following directions?

6. Does the child appear confused at times when listening to lengthy or challenging auditory information?

7. Does the child become easily distracted when involved in listening activities?

8. Does the child prefer small-group or one-to-one activities?

9. What subjects does the child like in school?

   What subjects does the child dislike?

10. How does the child do academically in school? Please specify present skills as well as past performance.

11. How is the child's self-esteem?

12. How are the child's social relationships?

Is there any other information that would be helpful to know?

Central Auditory Processing Disorder / Dorothy A. Kelly, D.A. / ISBN 0761631623

The Diagnostic Evaluation
(Representative only)

Speech-Language Evaluation as per
Possible Central Auditory Processing Dysfunction

Date:

Child's Name:

Date of Birth:

School:

Grade/Placement:

Date of Evaluation:

Address:

Referral Source/Reason for Evaluation:

Speech-Language Pathologist:

Background Information:

Tests and Assessment Tools Administered:

(continued)

Central Auditory Processing Disorder / Dorothy A. Kelly, D.A. / ISBN 0761631623

Reading Decoding Tool and Spelling Procedures:

Child's Auditory Processing Skills Profile—Parent's Observations:

**Behaviors in Children with Central Auditory Processing Disorders—
A Checklist for the Classroom Teacher:**

Language Sample:

Additional Assessment Procedures:

(continued)

Central Auditory Processing Disorder / Dorothy A. Kelly, D.A. / ISBN 0761631623

Interpretation of Results:

Scores will be discussed in terms of five major categories of central auditory processing skills which impact on academic and social settings. These categories are: auditory figure-ground, auditory memory, auditory discrimination, auditory cohesion, and auditory attention.

1. Auditory Figure-Ground Skills (the ability to screen out ambient or background noise distractions):

2. Auditory Memory Skills (the ability to recall a variety of auditorily sequenced units):

3. Auditory Discrimination Skills (the ability to note minor phonemic differences):

4. Auditory Cohesion Skills (the ability to employ higher-order cognitive/processing skills in a meaningful manner):

5. Auditory Attention (the ability to maintain attention purposely over an extended period of time):

Summary of Results:

Recommendations:

Speech-Language Pathologist

Central Auditory Processing Disorder / Dorothy A. Kelly, D.A. / ISBN 0761631623

Central Auditory Processing Progress Report

Child:

Date of Birth:

School District:

Grade/Placement:

Date:

Speech-Language Pathologist:

Updated Assessment Results:

Status of Progress:

Recommendations:

_____
Speech-Language Pathologist

PART THREE

Practical Suggestions for Parents, Teachers, and Students

Chapters 4, 5, and 6 are designed to provide practical, everyday information, strategies, and materials to students with CAPD and their parents and teachers.

The questions and answers on pages 89-90 may be used as part of an inservice presentation to teachers or for parent instruction.

Chapter 4, Suggestions for Parents, identifies possible behaviors at home, provides suggestions for Committee of Special Education meetings, and makes various communication suggestions.

Chapter 5, Suggestions for Teachers, provides practical identification and intervention advice and discusses placement options, among other matters.

Chapter 6, Suggestions for Students, offers a variety of materials designed to help the child become more aware of auditory experiences and learn to modify and organize them. Responsibility and active participation are encouraged throughout.

4

Suggestions for Parents

Questions and Answers for Parents and Teachers

1. What is central auditory processing disorder?

   Central auditory processing disorder (or dysfunction) is a condition in which the ability to interpret or process words and sounds is impaired in some way. Although the words or sounds are heard (through the ear), the auditory nervous system (beyond the ear going to the brain) does not process them.

2. How is central auditory processing disorder different from hearing loss?

   In hearing loss, hearing levels can be measured through audiometry or hearing testing. Based on the type and extent of the loss, they can be diagnosed. Some conditions respond well to hearing aids. But central auditory processing disorders are more "internal" than "external," and they cannot be measured by hearing tests alone or treated by ordinary hearing aids.

3. What causes central auditory processing disorders?

   Just as there are many types of CAPD, there are many causes. Some possible factors include changes in the blood vessels or nerves that serve the brain, and chronic otitis media (infection in the middle ear). CAPDs can occur in adults as well as in children, and the disorders can range from mild to severe.

4. What are some of the symptoms?

   The symptoms also vary. Some of the more common symptoms include inability to remember what is heard, problems in following directions, difficulty with background noises, and limited ability to listen. Any combination of symptoms can be present.

   (continued)

5. How does CAPD affect behavior?

    It's important to remember that a child with CAPD has not "chosen" to behave inappropriately. For example, the child does not fail to carry out directions on purpose. Most children don't recognize that they are not processing what they hear. The children simply find that as situations become difficult, they become frustrated and may respond by "acting out."

    The child may have other conditions, such as attention deficit disorder, along with the processing disorder. This makes it much more difficult to diagnose the problem.

6. How do central auditory processing disorders affect classroom performance?

    When we look at the various symptoms, we can see how they can affect the child's performance. For example, a child who has problems screening out background noise may not follow directions or be able to listen to a lecture in a noisy classroom. Often, just a few minor changes in the classroom can improve the listening environment for the child.

7. How do central auditory processing disorders affect behavior at home?

    A child who has problems with background noises, following directions in the classroom, or other processing difficulties will have the same problems at home. The listening environment can be changed at home as well as at school. Speakers can be taught strategies that will make it easier for the child to process what is heard.

8. What subjects are affected?

    When processing skills are poor, *all* subjects can be affected; but reading, spelling, writing, and vocabulary skills are affected most often. After repeated "failures" and much frustration, another problem sometimes develops. Some of these children begin to think of themselves as stupid or incompetent and may "turn off" to school.

9. Will the child "grow out of it"?

    Because CAPD is most likely a disorder of the auditory nervous system, the child will *not* simply grow out of it. But the child can learn strategies that will help in coping with difficult situations.

10. Can central auditory processing disorders be treated?

    Improvements often are possible in all the areas of processing. These children must be taught in a different way. Their auditory processing skills must be developed. They are tools to help the child function independently. The child must take active, ongoing responsibility in applying the new skills and strategies to everyday life.

Central Auditory Processing Disorder / Dorothy A. Kelly, D.A. / ISBN 0761631623

Symptoms Presented at Home

Children with central auditory processing disorders show problem behaviors at home as well as in school. Many of these behaviors are also present in other disorders, such as attention deficit disorder or learning disabilities.

A child with CAPD may have many of these symptoms:

1. Shows unusual reaction to sudden or loud sounds.

2. Has problems recalling names, dates, times, and other information.

3. Has difficulty identifying the source or location of a sound.

4. Has poor memory for numbers, letters, words, and other information that is heard.

5. Has difficulty following simple directions.

6. Has difficulty following complicated directions.

7. Has difficulty interpreting abstract information.

8. Has difficulty with dictated information.

9. Is easily distracted by noises.

10. Performs better in small groups.

11. Has difficulty with background noises.

12. Has poor musical abilities.

13. Sometimes appears confused.

14. Has difficulty with spelling.

15. Has difficulty with reading.

16. Has difficulty with word math problems.

17. Has poor self-esteem and few friends.

18. Has difficulty with written expression.

19. Has difficulty with directions that are to be carried out later.

20. Is unorganized and messy.

21. Has difficulty with appointments, routines, and chores.

22. Asks for statements to be repeated.

23. Confuses one sound for another.

24. Is slow to respond to questions or directions.

25. Gives inappropriate answers to simple questions.

26. Gives inappropriate responses in conversations.

27. Has a speech problem.

Central Auditory Processing Disorder / Dorothy A. Kelly, D.A. / ISBN 0761631623

Strategies That Help at Home

You can use many strategies to make your child's listening experiences more successful. Your child's speech-language pathologist will be able to tell you about other techniques that may be helpful.

Following Directions

Probably the most frequently occurring problem is not being able to follow directions. There are several reasons for this problem. Your child's problems may increase:

- When there is noise in the background, or
- When the direction is complicated, or
- When the direction is lengthy, or
- If the direction has to carried out some time later.

Observe your child's behavior carefully for several weeks. Notice how the child responds to various situations. When we recognize the cause of the child's problem, simple solutions often occur to us naturally. Here are two simple changes may make it easier for your child to process directions and finish a task.

- Reduce background noise. (For example, does your child have trouble following directions when the TV is on? Turn off the TV and try again.)
- Be sure your child is looking at you when you speak.

If your child's problems occur mainly when the directions are lengthy or complicated, find a better way to give directions.

- First, make eye contact with the child.
- Then speak at a slightly slower rate, with a little more expression in your voice.
- Use simpler, shorter sentences.
- Pause briefly between parts of the direction. For example, instead of saying, "Go upstairs and find your red sweater and put it in the clothes hamper," say, "Go upstairs. . . . Put your red sweater in the hamper."
- Ask the child to repeat the direction over and over in a low voice (or silently) until the task is finished.
- Another reminder is to say to the child, "Make a picture in your mind. See yourself going upstairs. See yourself getting your red sweater. Now see yourself putting it in the hamper."

Remembering Directions

Does your child have a problem remembering tasks that are to be done later? Strategies can help here, too.

- Begin by asking the child to carry out a simple task in five minutes. Then gradually increase the time to ten minutes, then thirty minutes, and so on.

(continued)

Central Auditory Processing Disorder / Dorothy A. Kelly, D.A. / ISBN 0761631623

- Ask your child, "How can we work together to help you remember the direction?" Some children write notes to themselves, or wear clothing items or markers (for example, putting stickers on their belts) to remind themselves.

- Wearing a watch helps the child build an awareness of time. It helps your child to develop a sense of schedules, appointments, and deadlines.

- And don't forget what a powerful model *you* are for your child when *you* are on time and organized.

Developing Better Habits

Encourage your child to develop these habits:

- Write down homework assignments.

- Do homework at a certain time every day, with the radio and TV off.

- Keep a neat desk and room.

- Plan what clothing to wear the next day.

- Finish regular chores around the house.

Changing the Listening Environment

Help your child to become aware of listening situations that might present problems. Encourage your child to do whatever is possible to improve the situation. For example, if the child is not able to see the speaker, the child could move closer. If a complicated direction is given while the TV is on, the child could ask to shut the TV off.

Changing Attitudes

The most important thing you can do is to encourage changes in your child's attitude.

- Help your child to think of himself or herself as an active member of a team who is involved in the *solution*—not just the *problem*.

- Help the child realize that the changes are being made for important reasons—not just for you, but for the child.

- Let the child make a *choice* about how much effort to make.

- Help the child to see that success is a worthwhile goal, and that when changes are *not* made, success will be limited.

These strategies are not cure-alls, but they can be used as tools to make day-to-day life run more smoothly. Remember that your child has not chosen to have these difficulties. With patience, encouragement, and understanding, your child can learn to work with the disability. Then self-esteem can grow, too!

Committee of Special Education Meetings—
Requests and Questions

Parents often have questions about the "what, how, when, and whys" of planning educational goals. Some of their questions are listed below. Your child's speech-language pathologist and other staff members can answer these and other questions you may have. Their answers will be based on your child's needs.

- What does central auditory processing involve?

- How does central auditory processing affect my child's classroom behavior?

- How was the diagnosis of central auditory processing disorder made? What assessments and tests were used to make the diagnosis? Are the tests norm-referenced?

- Please explain the goals you have set for my child. Why did you choose these goals at this particular time?

- How does each of these goals relate to classroom learning skills?

- In which classroom activities will the auditory trainer be used? Why? How will you gradually reduce my child's dependence on the auditory trainer?

- What changes will you make in the classroom to help my child become a better listener? (Different seating, working in small groups, and so on)

- What strategies or techniques will the teacher use in the classroom to help my child process better? How is the teacher being taught these procedures?

- What strategies or techniques can I use at home? How, when, and where will you teach them to me?

- How will my child be grouped in therapy? What are your reasons for that grouping?

- Do you plan to gradually reduce my child's therapy time? If so, when and why?

- What are my child's responsibilities in the process?

- Will my child be taught how to carry over the new skills from the therapy room to the classroom and everyday life?

- Where do you see my child in two years, in terms of classroom placement and necessary services?

- How will progress or therapy gains be measured?

- How will the speech-language pathologist and the teacher share their observations about my child's progress?

- How will the speech-language pathologist and I share observations about my child's progress?

- How often will my child be evaluated?

- How will my child's hearing be measured? How often?

- How do you plan to help my child improve self-esteem?

Resources for Parents

A variety of support and information is available to the parents of children with CAPD. These sources may be used "as needed." They include the following people.

Speech-Language Pathologist—A professional who has a key role in diagnosing your child's disorder. The person who will provide periodic evaluations, therapy services, and progress updates. A member of the Committee of Special Education team.

Audiologist—A professional who completes the child's initial audiology evaluation. If a hearing loss is found, the person who periodically evaluates hearing status and provides management services, if needed. The person who specifies type of auditory trainer, if needed.

Otolaryngologist—A medical physician, otherwise known as an "ear, nose, and throat doctor." May be involved in treatment of child's otitis media, including inserting pressure-equalizing tubes and prescribing medications.

Classroom or Resource-Room Teachers—Provide information about how the child with CAPD is applying strategies to academic and classroom tasks. Key members of the Committee of Special Education team. May provide frequent progress updates.

School Nurse—Provides regular auditory and visual screenings. Is a good source of information about changes in hearing in a child with chronic otitis media. Provides other medically-based information.

Parent Advocate—Serves on the Committee of Special Education. Is a support person for the parent. May voice concerns or raise questions about educational plans, placements, diagnoses, and other issues.

Other Parents—The speech-language pathologist may be able to provide names of other parents of children with central auditory processing disorder (with their permission) to share strategies, problem-solving techniques, and other information.

Special Education Parent-Teacher Associations—An organized group of interested parents, teachers, and professionals who meet regularly to share strategies, problem-solving techniques, and other information; they organize group efforts, when needed, to promote quality education for special education students.

Other Professionals—School administrators, psychologists, social workers, and others who provide support and information as needed.

American Speech-Language-Hearing Association—A professional organization that provides information on a variety of communication disorders, among other activities.
Address: 10801 Rockville Pike, Rockville, Maryland 20852
Telephone: 301-897-5700

Activities for Parents and Children

Many activities are designed to improve the child's ability to organize, categorize, remember, and carry on a conversation. These activities work best when they are done naturally during everyday situations at home.

The activities should never be thought of as "work" or "therapy." If you and your child aren't having fun, don't do them.

- At mealtime, include your child in family conversations. Encourage your child to talk about what happened in school and listen as family members talk about their experiences. Be sure your child is looking at the speaker's face. Turn off the TV and the radio, and eliminate as much background noise as possible. If your child has difficulty following a conversation or adding to it appropriately, recap the content by speaking in short sentences with much expression in your voice.

- Play games that require the players to use logic, strategies, and problem-solving. Spelling and vocabulary games are good. Games in which no one "loses" are best.

- Encourage the habit of making lists for a variety of purposes such as groceries, chores, and homework assignments. This helps to develop planning and organizational skills.

- Encourage your child to plan what to wear for the next day. Help the child to select clothes that are appropriate. Explain why some combinations may not match, and show your child other combinations that go well together. Let your child help select new clothes.

- Play the Telephone Game. (See page 141.)

- Play Simon Says. (See page 238.)

- Play the Traveling by Rocket Ship game (pages 234-236) and the Sound-It-Out Game (pages 237-238).

- Watch good television programs that last at least 1/2 hour and that involve characterizations and plot development. Watch the programs with your child. At the end of the program, talk with your child about opinions, logical solutions to problems posed, sequence of events, character flaws, poor choices made by characters, and alternative endings. Perhaps your child will want to write a brief summary of the events.

- Play games in the car. Encourage games that require the child to identify (for example, look for license plates from particular states or with particular letters or numbers). Answer and ask riddles, and sing silly songs.

(continued)

Central Auditory Processing Disorder / Dorothy A. Kelly, D.A. / ISBN 0761631623

Activities for Parents and Children (continued)

- Play memory games. Add-on games are excellent memory builders. For example:

  Parent: I went to the toy store and I bought an archery set.

  Child: I went to the toy store and I bought an archery set and a bike.

  Parent: I went to the toy store and I bought an archery set and a bike and a checkers game.

  Child: I went to the toy store and . . .

- "I Spy" games are good, too.

- Encourage your child to listen for words that give clues about the order of events. For example, words such as "now," "later," "after," and "before" provide information about time and sequence.

- Encourage your child to make a mental picture whenever possible. These images are helpful when recalling a conversation, direction, a phone number, or a homework assignment.

- Read stories to your child. After each page or two, ask the child to recap what was heard. At the end, ask your child to summarize the entire story.

Central Auditory Processing Disorder / Dorothy A. Kelly, D.A. / ISBN 0761631623

Miscellaneous Activities for Children

The following list of 20 words can serve as the basis for many activities, including:

- Word scrambles

- Finding all the little words within each larger word

- Syllable counting

- Spelling forward and backward

- Defining

- Categorizing

- Constructing sentences and paragraphs

- Alphabetizing

Can you and your child think of other activities?

Word List

1.	attention	11.	memory
2.	auditory	12.	monitor
3.	syllables	13.	note taking
4.	communication	14.	organization
5.	comprehension	15.	processing
6.	directions	16.	proofreading
7.	discrimination	17.	success
8.	figure-ground	18.	reasoning
9.	focusing	19.	strategies
10.	intonation	20.	listening

How Am I Doing?
A Checklist for Parents

Have I . . .

1. Limited background noises at home whenever possible?

2. Set up schedules with time for homework, telephone, TV, and fun?

3. Spoken in simple sentences with expression in my voice?

4. Kept ongoing contact with teachers and therapists?

5. Set up lists for my child's chores?

6. Modeled good behavior by keeping my own appointments on time?

7. Provided my child with an assignment pad, tape recorder, and other aids?

8. Praised my child's successes?

9. Made an effort to improve my child's self-esteem?

10. Encouraged my child to make choices, accept responsibilities, and use logic?

11. Presented a positive and realistic view of therapy and school experiences?

12. Used daily activities as opportunities to improve skills?

13. Used daily activities as opportunities to problem-solve, organize, categorize, predict, sequence, synthesize, and simplify?

14. Used daily experiences as opportunities to develop good habits and patterns?

15. Encouraged my child to set goals for himself or herself, rather than to achieve goals that I have set? (For example, does my child see the value of getting better grades in school?)

16. Encouraged my child to keep a clean room, neat work area, and organized clothes closet?

17. Provided my child with a quiet, distraction-free work area?

18. Worked with the other parent or close relative in my child's life to present a unified plan of goals, strategies, and praise?

19. Maintained mutual eye contact with my child when conversing?

20. Encouraged healthy habits such as eating good foods and getting enough sleep?

Child's Name:	
Parent's or Guardian's Name:	Date:

Child's Auditory Processing Skills Profile—
Parent's Observations

Please describe your child's listening behaviors at home. With the information you provide, your child's test results can be compared with the child's natural behavior.

Key:
A = Better than average skills or performance
B = Average skills or performance
C = Mild difficulty
D = Moderate difficulty
E = Severe difficulty
F = Do not know

Please indicate your child's performance when listening or processing:	A	B	C	D	E	F
1. In noisy settings						
2. Simple directions						
3. Complicated directions						
4. Over a period of time						
5. In settings with visual distractions						
6. Directions to be carried out later						
7. At a distance from the speaker						
8. Abstract or logic-based information						
9. Information produced loudly						
10. While feeling tired						
11. While looking at the speaker's face						
12. Lengthy conversations						

(continued)

13. Does your child have a history of ear infections (particularly from birth to age three)? If so, please explain. Describe any treatment.

14. Does your child appear to "hear" better on some days than on others? If so, please explain.

15. How does your child feel about school?

What subjects does your child like and dislike?

16. Is there any additional information that would be helpful?

Thank you

_____
Speech-Language Pathologist

5

Suggestions for Teachers

For the Classroom Teacher

Identifying children with central auditory processing disorders involves input from various team members, including the classroom teacher. Once the diagnosis has been confirmed and the particular nature of the disorder specified, accommodations may be made in the classroom. Many of these accommodations are simple modifications of the child's listening environment. These changes make your job easier as well as the child's.

Depending on the specific diagnosis and the child's progress in therapy, recommendations will vary. For example, if the child has an auditory figure-ground problem (difficulty screening out background noise), recommendations may be to increase one-to-one opportunities, seat the child toward the front of the room facing away from the window, and limit auditory distractions. In some cases, the child may be fitted temporarily with an auditory trainer. In this event, the child wears a headset and the teacher wears a microphone. The fitting audiologist and the speech-language pathologist will give specific recommendations about when and how much to use the trainer.

If the child has an auditory memory problem and has difficulty following directions, the teacher may simply modify the style used for presenting material. Sentences may be produced at a slightly slower rate, with slightly increased vocal volume, more expressive intonation, and clear facial expression and gestures. These suggestions aid the natural speech-reading process used by many children with CAPD. Also, the child will be able to respond to directions better if the words to be recalled are presented in "chunks." Make certain that the child is looking at you while you are speaking.

Directions can be naturally segmented with brief pauses before the next group of words is presented (for example, "Please open your math book . . . to page 109 . . . and do problems 10 through 15").

Another helpful technique to be used with children who have problems in following directions is to have the child say the direction over and over (either in low tones or silently) until the task is completed. Eye contact also is useful.

(continued)

Central Auditory Processing Disorder / Dorothy A. Kelly, D.A. / ISBN 0761631623

For the Classroom Teacher (continued)

Sometimes a child cannot seem to act on a direction at a later time (for example, "Do your spelling work at 10:00 a.m."). Reminder cues can help here. Some children write notes to themselves or are cued by visual reminders in the classroom.

Perhaps the child also has a latency problem (delay in processing time). In this event, simply allow more time to respond. If the child still has difficulty responding, repeat the direction and, if needed, rephrase it. For example, "Put your blue folders under your social studies book"; then, "Put your blue folders . . . under your social studies book"; then, "Take out your blue folders . . . and your social studies book." *(Pause for response.)* "Put the folders . . . under the book."

In terms of communication cues, *how* something is said is just as important as *what* is said. A child who has an auditory discrimination problem also may have problems with spelling, reading decoding, and following directions. Many classroom hassles can be avoided by simply identifying the problem and reacting appropriately. A child who seems confused by a direction may be interpreting it slightly differently. (For example, "Stack your books on the back shelf" may be "heard" as, "Pack your books on the rack shelf").

Because this child may be relying on context cues to a large extent, additional cues (such as using an expressive tone of voice, pointing, and other gestures) will make it easier for the child to comprehend.

If the child demonstrates an overall poor auditory attention span and is often distracted, modifications may help. Clear shorter exercises are called for until the child's focusing skills improve. The clearer the directions, the quieter the classroom, and the smaller the group, the longer the child may be able to attend. Visual cues also help the child to maintain focus (for example, an outline written on the chalkboard, or photocopied notes presented to the child in advance of a lecture). Don't overlook the psychological factor: The more successful the child feels in any task, the more likely that child will be motivated to attend.

A child who displays auditory cohesion or higher-order processing problems sometimes appears to lack "auditory logic." The child seems to be unable to interpret, to analyze, to associate, to categorize, to synthesize, and to conclude appropriately. This skill may be somewhat contingent upon other skills such as auditory attention.

As the child progresses in central auditory processing skills such as auditory memory and auditory attention, gains may be noted in auditory cohesion as well. Again, simple diagnosis of this problem area seems beneficial. Challenge the child in higher-order auditory tasks, but also break down the tasks into more manageable, sequenced units. For example, "Tell how a cow and a horse are alike and different" can be presented as, "Tell me about a cow. Tell me where a cow lives, what it eats, what it looks like, what kind of an animal it is, and anything else you can think of"; "Now, tell me about a horse"; "What did you name as the same for both the cow and the horse?"; "What things did you say were different about the cow and the horse?"

The classroom teacher also is asked to help the child with CAPD become more responsible and organized (for example, write down assignments, prepare for reports in advance, keep a clean desk and a neat notebook).

Children with CAPD are quite capable of learning. With knowledge and a few strategies, these children can succeed in the classroom.

Central Auditory Processing Disorder / Dorothy A. Kelly, D.A. / ISBN 0761631623

Symptoms Presented in the Classroom

Among children with CAPD, the range of severity and the variety of symptoms and classroom behaviors are wide. Many of the behaviors are also present in other disorders, such as attention deficit disorder or learning disabilities.

A child with CAPD may have many of these symptoms:

1. Shows unusual reaction to sudden and/or loud sounds.

2. Has problems recalling names, dates, times, and so on.

3. Has difficulty associating sound with its source or location.

4. Has poor auditory sequential memory for numbers, letters, words, and so on.

5. Has difficulty following simple directions.

6. Has difficulty following complicated directions.

7. Has difficulty interpreting abstract materials.

8. Has difficulty with dictated materials.

9. Is easily distracted by auditory stimuli.

10. Performs better in one-to-one settings.

11. Has difficulty with background noises.

12. Has very poor musical abilities.

13. Sometimes appears confused when auditory stimuli are presented.

14. Has difficulty with spelling.

15. Has difficulty with reading decoding.

16. Has difficulty with verbal math problems.

17. Has poor self-esteem.

18. Has difficulty with written expression; handwriting is poor.

19. Has difficulty with directions to be carried out later.

20. Is unorganized; has difficulty with appointments and routines.

21. Has difficulty with categorizations and associations.

22. Asks for repetitions of what has been said.

23. Confuses one sound for another.

24. Is slow to respond to questions or directions.

25. Gives inappropriate responses to simple questions.

26. Gives inappropriate responses in conversations.

27. Has a speech problem.

Central Auditory Processing Disorder / Dorothy A. Kelly, D.A. / ISBN 0761631623

Reading Questionnaire

For the Classroom Teacher and Speech-Language Pathologist

The following questions are designed to help clarify how the child's central auditory processing disorders impact on various tasks associated with reading. By identifying the specific effects upon reading, knowledge is gained regarding learning gaps and defective word attack strategies, as well as specific aspects of processing disorder. For example, a child with auditory discrimination problems is more likely to demonstrate vowel and consonant identification errors.

How a child reads has direct influence upon how the child spells and writes. By addressing defective strategies in reading and then supplying more effective strategies based on the child's central auditory processing needs, improvement may be seen in reading and reading-related tasks such as spelling and writing.

- -

Reading Questionnaire

Child's Name:		Date:	

Reading Aloud

Does the child:	Yes	No
Mark meaning with appropriate intonation?		
Vary rate according to meaning?		
Use appropriate vocal volume?		
Code accented syllables appropriately with intonation?		
Present some sort of variation or "style"?		
Occasionally look up at listeners?		

Timing

Does the child:	Yes	No
Allow more time between sentences than between words?		
Pause briefly at commas and other markers?		
Emphasize or give additional time to stressed or key words?		
Use an appropriate overall rate?		
Code accented syllables with elongated "time"?		

Vowel and Consonant Identification

Does the child:	Yes	No
Confuse short vowels?		
Confuse long vowels?		
Confuse stop consonants?		
Confuse consonant blends and clusters?		
Delete or reduce consonant blends and clusters?		
Reverse phoneme sequences?		

(continued)

Word Attack Skills

Is the child able to:	Yes	No
Correctly identify the number of syllables in a word?		
Blend separated syllables into a "whole" word?		
Break up "whole" words into syllables?		
Use syllable cues to spell words?		
Realize that suffixes, prefixes, and other word parts can be used in many different words?		
Produce all syllables in a word (not deleting weaker ones)?		

Phonics versus Sight Reading

Does the child:	Yes	No
Prefer learning new words through a "whole word" or sight approach?		
Have difficulty associating symbol with sound?		
Have difficulty applying decoding rules to new words?		
Display idiosyncratic word attack strategies?		
Display inconsistent word attack strategies?		
Appear to display few or no word attack strategies?		
Demonstrate a clear aversion to reading?		
Did the child acquire reading skills later than peers?		

Reading Comprehension

Does the child:	Yes	No
Seem to lose track of position on the page when reading?		
Seem to lose track of the theme or train of thought of the passage being read?		
Fail to make adequate interpretations?		
Fail to be able to summarize what was read?		
Succeed more with concrete questions?		
Misunderstand abstract vocabulary?		
Get "tired" quickly from reading?		

Can you provide any additional information regarding strategies or gaps?

Central Auditory Processing Disorder / Dorothy A. Kelly, D.A. / ISBN 0761631623

Read-Aloud Passage

The passage below is not meant to be an assessment tool for reading levels. It is designed to present a relatively low-challenge opportunity to observe the child's oral reading difficulties that may provide insight into central auditory processing problems.

Read-Aloud Passage

Name:

Date:

Teacher/Speech-Language Pathologist:

It was Kevin's first day at school. Not only was it his first day, it was also his first day in a new school. His family had just moved to New York City from Kansas, and he was scared. He had heard so many things about New York, many of them less than positive. He was afraid the kids would make fun of his accent. He was afraid that he didn't have the right clothes and that the other kids would all be smarter. As he opened his classroom door for the first time, he wished he could just evaporate into the air.
What happened next came as a total surprise!

Comments:

Additional Strategies

Because central auditory processing disorder often involves a variety of language-learning difficulties, procedures that provide additional means of reinforcing, defining, clarifying, and organizing language tasks are beneficial. When those procedures also allow the child to anticipate or predict outcomes or sequences, expectations are more likely to be met. Use of strategies also helps to reduce frustration for both the teacher and student.

The following strategies were offered by Leverett and Diefendorf (1992) for teachers working with students with language deficiencies. The techniques also have applications for students with CAPD.

Marginal Gloss—Glosses are notes written to students by the teacher in the margins of reading materials. These notes provide explanations and definitions of difficult materials. The teacher may also underline key concepts or vocabulary within the text itself.

Vocabulary Guide—Guides provide explanations of difficult terms written at the student's level. Words can be broken down into syllables with space allowed for brief writing tasks. Location or page number information is provided.

Advance Organizer—Vocabulary and concepts of reading assignments that are potentially confusing may be summarized in a simpler, introductory paragraph. This material is given to the student in advance.

Structured Overview—The child's present knowledge is combined with new information (including vocabulary), to be read in a flow chart or branching diagram.

Attribute/Classification Activities—Common and uncommon objects are brought into the classroom. The group categorizes their characteristics and lists them in chart form.

These techniques may be helpful to the regular classroom teacher who has a student with CAPD.

1. Have the student seated preferentially as directed. (See page 111.)

2. Have the student look at the speaker's face.

3. Limit background distractions of all kinds.

4. Present directions in short, concrete segments, with visual cues.

5. Rephrase directions, allowing extra time for response.

6. Code utterances with slightly louder volume, slightly slowed rate, and expressive intonation. The "melody" in speech provides additional communication cues.

7. Use as many natural and expressive gestures and facial expressions as possible.

8. Encourage students to work with a "buddy" or peer tutor when feasible.

(continued)

Central Auditory Processing Disorder / Dorothy A. Kelly, D.A. / ISBN 0761631623

Additional Strategies (continued)

9. Ask the student to restate concepts and directions as they were interpreted. Do this without singling out the student with CAPD.

10. Write assignments on the chalkboard. Have the students immediately copy the assignments into a homework pad. Just before the end of the day, ask students to locate their homework pads and any necessary materials to be taken home.

11. Allow tape recorders if they are helpful to the student.

12. Maintain structure and schedules as much as possible.

13. Relate new information and concepts to previously acquired information whenever possible.

14. Use demonstrations whenever possible; encourage hands-on activities.

15. Provide "quiet" areas in the classroom where concentration may be easier to maintain.

16. Preview materials to be presented, using a variety of media.

17. Summarize materials. Restate concepts, using simpler, more concrete terms.

18. Encourage an auditory awareness of voices, sounds, and words (for example, syllable parts in words, accent points, pitch changes in voices, volume changes, melodies or intonation in speech, and so on).

19. Build an awareness of word families, root bases, and rhyming words.

20. Segment complicated directions into parts, allowing time in between for processing.

21. Encourage auditory logic when possible (for example, "It couldn't be _____ because we heard the words _____. What is it then most likely?").

22. Classify, organize, categorize, outline, and summarize whenever possible. Provide varied and repeated opportunities with the same concepts and materials.

23. Demonstrate and encourage proofreading aloud of written expression. Grammatical, punctuation, and spelling errors may be more easily identified. The "sense" of the writing is more easily determined when read aloud.

24. Build students' self-esteem at every opportunity.

25. Involve the parents and other staff members in applying similar techniques and strategies.

Central Auditory Processing Disorder / Dorothy A. Kelly, D.A. / ISBN 0761631623

Preferential Seating

The diagrams below illustrate the most advantageous seating placements within the classroom for the student with CAPD.

Generally, seat the child toward the front of the room, with clear visual access to both the teacher and chalkboard area, and with back to the window area. Although not "hearing impaired," the child with CAPD may speech-read far more than is realized. Be aware of possible glare from fluorescent lighting, which may be harsh.

These modifications provide maximum opportunity to "read" the entire communication picture, including visual, gestural, and auditory cues. They also attempt to reduce the number of extraneous distractions.

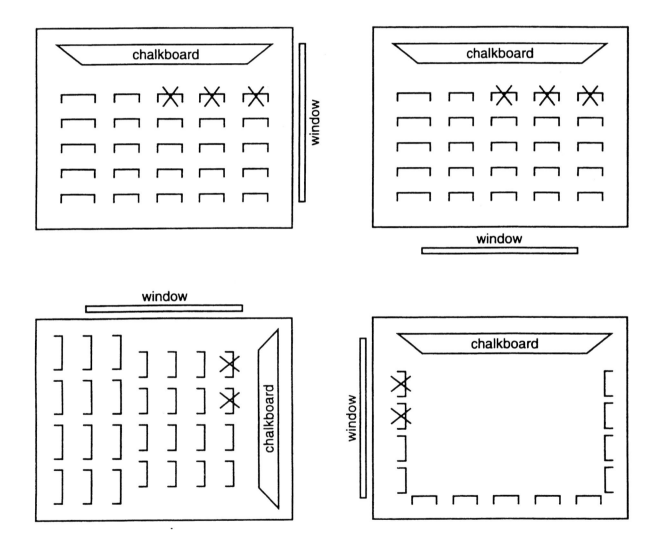

Monthly Progress Summary

To:	_____ , Classroom Teacher/Resource Room Teacher
From:	_____ , Speech-Language Pathologist
Month:	
Student:	
Date:	

Please rate this student's progress in each of the checked areas of central auditory processing. Include any miscellaneous comments that you feel would be helpful. Thank you.

	Excellent	Good	Fair	Poor	Not Sure
Overall auditory attention					
Auditory figure-ground					
Following directions					
Auditory memory					
Auditory discrimination					
Auditory cohesion					

Related Tasks:

Spelling					
Writing					
Reading decoding					
Other					

Comments:

Central Auditory Processing Disorder / Dorothy A. Kelly, D.A. / ISBN 0761631623

Inservice for Teachers

The following outline may be used by speech-language pathologists when providing inservice presentations to teachers and other staff members on central auditory processing disorders. It reflects the need to provide foundation information and basic vocabulary as well as to identify applications to classroom subject areas and tasks.

Central Auditory Processing Disorders

I. Hearing is different from listening.

   A. Hearing is a mechanical process, while listening is an active perceptual process involving *meaning* and *comprehension*. A child can have normal hearing and impaired perception. Whereas hearing is "ear-based," central auditory processing is based beyond the ear, somewhere in the auditory nervous system.

   B. Auditory processing skills are numerous. They include auditory memory, auditory figure-ground, auditory discrimination, and auditory attention.

   C. Perceptual development involves the interaction of cognitive, biological, developmental, and experiential factors. CAPDs are not functions of intelligence, personality, or volition.

   D. Several central auditory perceptual or processing skills, such as auditory figure-ground and auditory memory, develop over time. For example, auditory figure-ground skills appear to stabilize at approximately age six or seven in normally progressing children. Auditory memory skills develop at approximately the following rate (Terman and Merrill 1960).

Chronological age	Number of units recalled
2.5 yrs.	2
3 yrs.	3
4.5 yrs.	4
7 yrs.	5
10 yrs.	6
Adult	7

   E. A history of chronic otitis media, lesions in the auditory nervous system, and other factors may negatively affect central processing development. Symptoms may be mild to severe and may evolve or change over time. However, central auditory processing disorders often are not ever completely remediated.

(continuted)

Central Auditory Processing Disorders (continued)

II. Central auditory processing disorders are varied.

    A. Central auditory processing disorders may exist as primary or secondary conditions in children or adults. Many children with learning disabilities and attention deficit disorder also exhibit central auditory processing disorders.

    B. Children with CAPDs may exhibit a wide variety of deficits in varying degrees and combinations. Each case is different, although auditory memory, auditory figure-ground, auditory discrimination, and auditory attention problems are fairly common.

III. Central auditory processing disorders may impact upon classroom performance.

    A. CAPDs may affect spelling, reading, writing, following directions, and other skills. Overall attention, distractibility, ability to screen out background noises, and peer interactions also may be influenced.

    B. Intervention may take several forms and involve auditory trainers, audiotaped programs, and other therapy options.

    C. Strategies may be used by the classroom teacher, the parents, and the child to make processing more productive. Classroom modifications are important. The child must be an active participant in recognizing difficult listening environments and applying strategies.

    D. Strategies may be acquired that make spelling, reading decoding, and writing easier.

    E. With appropriate identification and intervention, the academic picture is never bleak and is usually manageable. Appropriate intervention often produces a very positive ripple effect in terms of the child's self-esteem and overall behavior.

Placement Options

Because the CAPD population is heterogeneous in nature, a wide variety of placement options exist. Although particular disorders do not necessarily require specific placements, certain general guidelines and issues may apply.

The following list of educational placements and service options represents a partial listing of plans available to students with CAPD.

Mainstreaming—The student is able to participate in one or more subjects within regular classroom settings.

- Depends on the particular child's diagnostic profile, the subjects involved, and the nature of the classroom setting (degree of ambient noise, numbers of students in room, degree of structure, and so on).

- May be possible for students with auditory discrimination, auditory memory, auditory figure-ground (if setting is quiet and structured), and/or auditory cohesion difficulties.

Resource Room—The student is placed within a regular classroom and goes out to the resource room for special subjects or for tutorial purposes.

- May be helpful for the child with academic and/or language disorders.

- May be helpful for the child with additional disorders such as executive dysfunction, attention deficit disorder, and learning disabilities.

- Use in conjunction with speech-language services.

- May be helpful for a child with auditory memory, auditory figure-ground, auditory attention, auditory cohesion, and/or auditory discrimination difficulties.

Regular Placement with Support Services—The student is placed within a regular classroom and receives special services usually outside the classroom (known as pull-out).

- May be helpful for children who need foundation skills within the therapy room before transitioning into the classroom.

- May be helpful for children who would benefit from small-group stimulation.

- May be helpful in the beginning stages of intervention for children with auditory figure-ground difficulties.

Inclusion—Also known as transdisciplinary, curriculum-based, interdisciplinary, integrated, or classroom-based services. Students with special needs remain within a regular classroom. They receive direct support services within the classroom itself or other natural environments.

- For students in the beginning or intermediate stages of intervention for auditory figure-ground therapy, inclusion probably presents problems due to the increased levels of distractions.

(continued)

Central Auditory Processing Disorder / Dorothy A. Kelly, D.A. / ISBN 0761631623

- For children with auditory attention difficulties in all contexts: Probably presents problems except when the specialist is deskside.

- For children with executive dysfunction difficulties: Probably is helpful.

- For children with auditory memory, auditory discrimination, and auditory cohesion difficulties: Probably is helpful only when the specialist is deskside.

Consultant Teacher Model—Also known as collaborative consultation; may be applied to different classroom settings.

A specialist works in an indirect manner on a regular basis; consults with classroom teacher and others; monitors student's progress and problems of the student.

- For students in the transition phase of intervention where skills are to be applied to academic and social tasks: May be helpful.

- For the classroom teacher: May be helpful in terms of modifying listening environment, presentation styles, reading strategies, and so on.

- May be part of a comprehensive school program in which the speech-language consultant identifies students at risk for CAPDs.

Self-contained Program—For the majority of the school day, students remain in a special class with a lower student-to-teacher ratio.

- May be necessary on a temporary or longer basis for very involved children with complicating diagnoses.

- The speech-language pathologist may work within the classroom itself for much of the day.

Combination Model—Allows the Committee of Special Education team to structure any combination of these models, depending upon the needs of the student.

- Is helpful to all CAPD children at various points in the intervention process. Needs will change according to individuals, challenges, and progress.

Central Auditory Processing Disorder / Dorothy A. Kelly, D.A. / ISBN 0761631623

Child's Name:	Grade:
Teacher's Name:	Date:

Child's Auditory Processing Skills Profile—
Teacher's Observations

Diagnosis of central auditory processing dysfunction depends on many tests and observations, of which the following checklist is a small part.

Some of these behaviors may be observed in the "average" child as well as in children with other diagnoses.

The child:	Yes	No	Not Sure
1. Has difficulty following immediate directions.			
2. Has difficulty following delayed directions.			
3. Has difficulty maintaining auditory attention or focus.			
4. Has a poor memory span for numbers, words, sounds, and so on.			
5. Has difficulty with written dictation.			
6. Has difficulty with spelling words that are spelled the way they sound.			
7. Has difficulty with spelling words that are not spelled the way they sound.			
8. Has difficulty with sounding out or decoding reading words.			
9. Has extraordinary problems in learning a foreign language.			
10. Has extraordinary problems in learning phonics.			
11. Has an articulation or phonology problem.			
12. Has difficulty localizing a sound source.			
13. Has difficulty processing information in noisy settings.			
14. Has difficulty discriminating between similar sounds and/or similar-sounding words.			
15. Has apparent intonation differences in speech (monotone, high-pitched style, and so on).			
16. Does not seem to infer emotional status from speaker's tone of voice.			
17. Is unorganized or forgetful.			
18. Does not apply auditory logic consistently (for example, "Don't knock on the door if you see it's closed").			

(continued)

The child:	Yes	No	Not Sure
19. Has difficulty participating in lengthy or in-depth conversations.			
20. Has difficulty with categorizations, analogies, making inferences.			
21. Frequently needs clarification of oral directions.			
22. Frequently asks, "What?"			
23. Has a history of frequent ear infections.			
24. Shows excessive reaction to sudden or loud noises.			
25. Is very distractible.			
26. Appears to learn more efficiently through the visual mode.			
27. Has unusually poor music skills.			
28. Has poor receptive and/or expressive language skills; has difficulty with written expression; handwriting is poor.			
29. Has difficulty remembering specifics of conversations, dialogues, and so on.			

Is there anything else that you feel would be helpful to know?

Thank you.

_____

Speech-Language Pathologist

Copyright © 1995 by Communication Skill Builders, a division of The Psychological Corporation / All rights reserved / 1-800-228-0752

Central Auditory Processing Disorder / Dorothy A. Kelly, D.A. / ISBN 0761631623

6

Suggestions for Students

Identify and Develop Your Talents

You are a very unique and talented person. If you don't already know what your strengths and talents are, ask yourself the following questions. Then spend some enjoyable time each day developing your talent.

Am I good at:

1. sports?
2. drawing?
3. other forms of art?
4. writing stories?
5. fixing things?
6. building things?
7. painting?
8. babysitting?
9. telling jokes?
10. bike riding?
11. writing poems?
12. computers?
13. computer games?
14. other games?
15. singing?
16. dancing?
17. acting?
18. decorating?
19. fixing hair?
20. baking?
21. cleaning?
22. cheering people up?
23. taking care of pets?
24. helping around the house?
25. _____?
26. _____?

Central Auditory Processing Disorder / Dorothy A. Kelly, D.A. / ISBN 0761631623

Self-Affirmations

Self-esteem—feeling good about yourself—is important for everyone. A positive attitude about yourself quickens your progress.

Hang these pages on the wall in your room. Begin each day by saying one or two of these "good thoughts." Think about them throughout the day.

This is not a chore or a homework assignment. It is something that's good for you. You deserve the benefits from doing it. It's part of the whole process of looking at the challenges in your life from a new perspective.

Think of another "good thought" that would really work for you. *YOU* are the expert on you. What do you think?

Self-Affirmations

1. I am a terrific person.

2. I am bright and talented.

3. I feel very good about myself.

4. I can do well.

5. I enjoy the positive strokes my parents and teachers give me when I do well.

6. I am in control of what I do in school and at home.

7. Although grades are important, *I am not my grades*. I am a worthwhile, terrific person even if I have some school problems sometimes.

8. I can make changes in my listening surroundings that make listening easier for me.

9. When I make changes in my listening surroundings, it has nothing to do with how smart I am.

10. Many people have the same challenges as mine.

11. I make progress in my goals when I identify them and take an active part in dealing with them.

12. Many famous and successful adults had similar challenges when they were younger.

13. I like myself no matter what—and with good reason!

14. I choose to make changes. I choose to be more successful. My attitude directly affects my choices throughout the day.

15. Today is a brand-new day. Changes can begin right now.

16. How I did last year in school has nothing to do with how well I can do in school today.

17. Nobody is perfect. It's important to do my best, but I don't need to be perfect.

18. I am very proud of myself. I like who I am as a person.

19. Everyone is different. Many bright and talented people have had to learn some strategies in order to do well. They "chose" to learn about and use these strategies.

20. Mom and Dad (or _____) are proud of me. They are even more proud now that I've made the choice to succeed.

Student Notes

These facts are critical to success in therapy.

Use these facts to prepare for the quiz that follows on pages 124-125.

1. Listening is different from hearing.

2. People with normal hearing speech-read more than they realize.

3. Watching the speaker's face often makes understanding easier.

4. It is easier to adjust to background sound that is always the same (for example, the air conditioner sound) than to sound that changes (for example, music).

5. Women's and children's voices are usually more expressive than men's voices.

6. People use their eyes, ears, and situational cues in conversations.

7. Listening requires active participation and responsibility.

8. Auditory processing is ongoing. It involves constant use of skills and strategies in everyday tasks.

9. Skills such as auditory discrimination and memory directly affect the ability to follow directions.

10. It is possible to change listening environments (for example, a noisy classroom).

11. It is important to identify listening environments as good or poor. Then changes can be made and listening strategies applied.

12. The best place to sit in the classroom is toward the front, facing away from the window, with a direct view of the teacher's face.

13. Auditory processing skills develop at different rates in different people. It is never too late to improve them.

14. Auditory processing skills have a strong relationship to spelling, reading, speaking, and language skills.

15. Strategies such as "chunking" (recalling words in groups), repeating silently, and repeating in a low voice can be used for as long as needed to improve processing skills.

16. The student must "choose" to be successful. The student must see the value in doing well in the classroom as well as in other places.

17. Very bright children sometimes have problems with auditory processing. Problems are far more frequent than are commonly known.

(continued)

18. Information about conversations can be obtained from the words that are spoken as well as the manner in which they are said. Facial expressions, body language, and gestures provide additional information.

19. Spelling and reading skills may be improved by using syllabication skills (that is, noting numbers of syllables in words and accent points).

20. By writing down homework assignments and appointments, by keeping a neat desk and notebook, and by thinking of other ways of "getting organized," home and school life can improve.

Central Auditory Processing Disorder / Dorothy A. Kelly, D.A. / ISBN 0761631623

Name:	
Grade:	Date:

Student Quiz

Circle **T** for True or **F** for False.

1.	Listening is not different from hearing.	**T**	**F**
2.	People with normal hearing speech-read more than they realize.	**T**	**F**
3.	Watching the speaker's face often makes understanding easier.	**T**	**F**
4.	It is not easier to adjust to background sound that is always the same (for example, the air conditioner sound) than to sound that changes (for example, music).	**T**	**F**
5.	Women's and children's voices usually are not more expressive than men's voices.	**T**	**F**
6.	People use their eyes, ears, and situational cues in conversation.	**T**	**F**
7.	Listening requires active participation and responsibility.	**T**	**F**
8.	Auditory processing is ongoing. It involves constant use of skills and strategies in everyday tasks.	**T**	**F**
9.	Skills such as auditory discrimination and memory directly affect the ability to follow directions.	**T**	**F**
10.	It is not possible to change listening environments (for example, a noisy classroom).	**T**	**F**
11.	It is important to identify listening environments as good or poor so that changes can be made and listening strategies applied.	**T**	**F**
12.	The best place to sit in the classroom is toward the front, facing away from the window, with a direct view of the teacher's face.	**T**	**F**
13.	Auditory processing skills develop at different rates in different people. It is never too late to improve them.	**T**	**F**
14.	Auditory processing skills have little to do with spelling, reading, speaking, and language skills.	**T**	**F**
15.	Strategies such as "chunking," repeating silently, and repeating in a low voice can be used for as long as needed to improve processing skills.	**T**	**F**

(continued)

Central Auditory Processing Disorder / Dorothy A. Kelly, D.A. / ISBN 0761631623

16. The student must "choose" to be successful. The student must see the value in doing well in the classroom as well as in other places. **T F**

17. Very bright children sometimes have problems with auditory processing. Problems are far more frequent than are commonly known. **T F**

18. Information about conversations cannot be obtained from the words that are spoken as well as the manner in which they are said. Facial expressions, body language, and gestures do not provide additional information. **T F**

19. Spelling and reading skills are not improved by applying syllabication skills (that is, noting numbers of syllables in words and accent points). **T F**

20. By writing down homework assignments and appointments, by keeping a neat desk and notebook, and by thinking of other ways of "getting organized," home and school life can improve. **T F**

Central Auditory Processing Disorder / Dorothy A. Kelly, D.A. / ISBN 0761631623

| Name: | | | | | | | | | Grade: | |

How Am I Doing?
A Checklist for Students

Use this chart to check your progress at the end of each month.
Use the results to plan your goals for the next month.

Answer only the questions that relate to your program.

This information does not have to be shared with anyone.

Key:
+ More than last month
– Less than last month
= Same as last month
? Not sure

Skill	Months									
	Sept.	Oct.	Nov.	Dec.	Jan.	Feb.	March	April	May	June
Following directions at home										
Following directions at school										
Ignoring background noises										
Changing the listening surroundings (for example, moving my seat)										
Remembering chores and appointments										
Remembering homework assignments										
Keeping a neat desk										
Keeping neat and organized notebooks										
Preparing ahead for long-term assignments										
Using strategies and techniques										
Using self-affirmations										
Improving spelling skills										
Improving reading decoding skills										
Improving reading comprehension										
Wearing a watch										

What can I do this month to improve my performance?

Strategies for School Tasks

1. Check your work. Use the strategy of repeating directions to yourself silently or in a low voice.

2. Ask for more information. Ask the teacher to repeat directions in another way. Ask for answers to particular questions.

3. Follow directions exactly. Know what you are to do before you start doing anything. Repeat the steps to yourself silently or in a low voice as you do the job.

4. Auditory imagery—Make a picture in your mind. See yourself carrying out the job. This strategy is helpful with verbal math problems. (For example, imagine these scenes: "If you bought five pieces of gum for 50 cents each, how much did you spend? If you gave the cashier a $5 bill, how much change would you get back?")

5. Take accurate notes. Use note-taking strategies. (See page 161.) This is helpful for tests, written assignments, and other tasks.

6. Be organized. Keep your desk neat. Keep a weekly calendar (see page 132) and a homework planner (see pages 133-134). Prepare for long-term assignments ahead of time.

7. Break down complicated jobs or directions into simple parts. For example, your mother says, "If it is raining, wear your blue raincoat. Otherwise, wear your red sweatshirt." Break this down in your mind. Ask yourself, "Is it raining? No. So I'll wear my red sweatshirt."

8. Syllabication—Say the word to yourself silently or in a low voice. Count the number of syllables in a word by "hearing" the changes in your voice, the length of the syllable, and how loud the syllable is. This strategy is helpful in spelling, reading, and writing tasks.

9. During a lecture, take notes. As soon as possible after the lecture, write the most important facts. Use your notes to help you write the summary of what you have heard.

10. Self-evaluation—Ask yourself these questions:

    What am I being asked to do?

    Do I know how to do it?

    Do I have everything that I need?

    Am I doing it in the most efficient manner?

    Have I accomplished what I was supposed to do?

    What am I supposed to do when I have finished?

Strategies for Change in the Classroom

1. Sit in the right place. Sit toward the front of the room or near the chalkboard with your back to the windows. Make sure you can see the teacher.

2. Limit extra movements. Do not chew gum, fidget, talk to your neighbor, look out the window, or otherwise distract yourself. Extra movements drain away the energy you need for your listening job.

3. Use a tape recorder. Tape long lectures. Take notes, and write a summary as soon as possible.

4. Choose to work in a small group or with a single partner whenever possible. It will be easier to understand information, and there will be fewer distractions.

5. If you have an auditory trainer, use it exactly as your speech-language pathologist has taught you.

6. Reduce background noise. Identify noisy settings. Whenever possible, ask people to lower their voices, talk one at a time, shut off the television or radio, or reduce the noise that is causing the problem.

7. Speech-reading—Look at the speaker's face. Learn to "read" the extra clues the speaker gives (facial expressions, tone of voice, gestures, and so on).

8. Use clues from the listening surroundings and routines, and guess. (For example, "It's 9:00 Friday morning. My teacher is probably going to tell us about the spelling test soon"; or, "She can't be talking about the Social Studies project. I heard the word protractor, and we usually do math after lunch. She's probably talking about a math project.")

9. Use the Buddy System. Find a friend in class that you work well with, someone you can ask to sometimes repeat directions and information for you, someone you can share your special skills with (for example, perhaps you are a better artist and can help your friend with book report covers).

10. Get organized. Write down assignments immediately. Keep a neat desk and notebook. Return your library books on time. Study and plan assignments ahead of time. Wear a watch.

Preparing for Spelling Tests

Make an audiotape recording of the spelling list. Follow these steps:

1. Read the list aloud as if you were the teacher giving the test to the class. Stop for about 15 seconds in between each word. For example, "Spell *successful* . . . Spell *remember* . . . Spell . . ."

2. Practice each word by looking at it and spelling it aloud. Listen to your own voice. Listen to the various syllable cues. Do this as many times as you need.

3. Play back the tape recording of your own voice reading the spelling list. As you hear your voice, spell the words out loud. Do this as many times as you need.

4. Listen to the tape recording again, and pretend you are taking the test. This time, write each word, just as you will have to do in the classroom. Do this as many times as you need.

Central Auditory Processing Disorder / Dorothy A. Kelly, D.A. / ISBN 0761631623

Getting Organized on School Days

In the Morning

Did I—

- Brush my teeth?
- Take my vitamin pills?
- Put my homework and books in my backpack?
- Take my lunch?
- Turn off my bedroom light?
- Straighten my bed?
- Pick up any towels or clothes from the floor?
- Put on my watch?
- Do my morning chores?

- _____

- _____

In the Afternoon

Did I—

- Put my backpack on my desk or work area?
- Give Mom or Dad any notices from school?
- Show Mom or Dad any graded tests?
- Hang up my jacket or sweater?
- Check my homework pad and make a homework plan?
- Do my afternoon chores?
- Start my homework by _____ P.M.?

- _____

- _____

(continued)

In the Evening

Did I—

- Finish my homework?
- Lay out my clothes for tomorrow?
- Set up my backpack?
- Make my lunch for tomorrow?
- Take my shower?
- Write down any needed reminders for tomorrow?
- Do my evening chores?
- Set my alarm clock for tomorrow morning?

- _____

- _____

Central Auditory Processing Disorder / Dorothy A. Kelly, D.A. / ISBN 0761631623

Weekly Calendar

Name:			Week of:	

	Chores	Homework	Appointments
Sunday			
Monday			
Tuesday			
Wednesday			
Thursday			
Friday			
Saturday			

Central Auditory Processing Disorder / Dorothy A. Kelly, D.A. / ISBN 0761631623

Homework Planner
Primary (Elementary Grades)

Week:

	Language Arts	Math	Science	Social Studies	Other	Other	Other
Monday							
Tuesday							
Wednesday							
Thursday							
Friday							

Week:

	Language Arts	Math	Science	Social Studies	Other	Other	Other
Monday							
Tuesday							
Wednesday							
Thursday							
Friday							

Homework Planner
Secondary (Junior High or High School)

Week:

	English	Science	Foreign Language	Social Studies	Math	Other	Other
Monday							
Tuesday							
Wednesday							
Thursday							
Friday							

Week:

	English	Science	Foreign Language	Social Studies	Math	Other	Other
Monday							
Tuesday							
Wednesday							
Thursday							
Friday							

Central Auditory Processing Disorder / Dorothy A. Kelly, D.A. / ISBN 0761631623

PART FOUR

Intervention and Remediation

Part Four is designed to provide the clinician with practical information, strategies, and materials useful for intervention with students who have central auditory processing disorders.

Chapter 7, Therapy Focuses and Strategies, offers insights regarding each of the auditory processing skill areas, provides techniques for remediation and classroom accommodation, and identifies individual education program (IEP) goals, among other information.

Chapter 8, Therapy Materials, provides strategies and techniques for strengthening auditory memory, following directions, auditory discrimination, and other areas.

7

Therapy Focuses and Strategies

CAPD Intervention in Summary Form

The following outline reflects key focuses for the central auditory processing intervention program described in this book.

It is less important to use particular materials or tests than it is to examine and address all possible areas of disorder in a comprehensive and competent manner and to understand how various disorders impact upon the child's life.

The materials presented in chapter 8 are representative rather than comprehensive in nature.

Successful intervention requires a blending of three key areas: psychology, therapy, and academic applications. These areas of concern are interdependent and mutually influential. Without an appropriate psychological set, the child is not likely to respond well to therapy; this in turn will limit the application of skills in the classroom. Thus, a fundamental beginning to all therapy programs, no matter what the particular areas of therapy focus, is to establish the appropriate psychological set.

This state of mind is one in which the child feels empowered—able to identify and modify listening experiences. The child further identifies talents and strengths and feels a part of a team effort that will please not only parents and teachers but the child as well.

1. Psychological Component

   • Self-affirmations

   • Identification of strengths

   • Correlations of weaker areas to specific social and academic difficulties

   • Concept of "team" approach

   • Support system involving parents, teachers, and others

   • Building a vested interest in the outcome of therapy; the child has input, controls, and the realization of goals to look forward to

2. Therapeutic Component

- Specific strategies to identify and modify the listening environment and the quality of listening experiences

- Habilitation (or rehabilitation) of:

  Auditory memory

  Auditory discrimination

  Auditory figure-ground

  Auditory attention

  Auditory cohesion

- Strategies to organize, predict, simplify, synthesize, interpret, and so on

- Application of skills to real-life settings and tasks in the classroom and home

- Responsibilities at home and in school

3. Academic Component

- Application of skills to reading, spelling, speaking, expressive writing, receptive comprehension, vocabulary, concept acquisitions, and other tasks

On Improving Auditory Memory Skills

Auditory memory skills involve the recall of auditory information in a variety of forms, including digits, unrelated words, letters, sentences, and other units. *Auditory sequential memory* involves a more demanding skill of recalling such units in specific orders, as opposed to recalling all the units but not necessarily in correct order. There also is immediate and delayed recall, the latter term implying an ability to defer response of some kind.

Thus, auditory memory skills may be placed into hierarchical forms, with immediate recall of shorter sequences being less challenging than delayed recall of longer sequences. The ability to recall sequences does not necessarily indicate that a child then can carry out directions—and especially complicated or deferred directions. These skills appear to be related, although not exactly the same in nature. The speech-language pathologist must be sensitive to such differences, especially when complicating problems exist (for example, auditory figure-ground difficulties).

The first task is to identify the specific areas of memory deficit and implement a program that proceeds hierarchically. The ability to carry out immediate and delayed complex directions in noise is the most challenging and probably should be addressed in the final stages of a program. In most cases, therapy should begin in the therapy room and progress to the classroom.

There are various patterns of memory deficit. Perhaps one child recalls only the beginning and middle parts of a sequence and tends to omit the final elements, while another child may recall only the last parts in a sequence. While not all children exhibit patterns, when a pattern is identified problem areas may be emphasized by varying rate, rhythm, and intonation cues. In this way, the child is provided with additional means to retain the information. Ask the child to visualize the sequence as it is heard and imagine writing it on the chalkboard. Some children like to trace the sequence with a finger on the knee as it is heard.

The issue of whether memory training should involve visual cues (that is, looking at the speaker's face) may involve a judgment call depending on the child's profile and needs. However, there is very little evidence that straight memory training of lengthening units (words, numbers, sentences) is effective. "More" is not necessarily helpful—especially if "more" involves mere repetition. (Perhaps this notion relates broadly to the "quantitative" versus "qualitative" issue noted earlier.) If repetition were all that were needed, the child probably would have not had an auditory memory problem to begin with. For whatever reasons, this child has not profited from repeated auditory experiences as an aid in extending memory. This child must be provided with additional cues to retain information. Therefore, it makes more sense to allow the child to exploit visual cues from the beginning of therapy, because that is most natural. Incorporating "difficult-to-view" contexts into the program (for example, viewing speakers from the side or from a distance) will increase the level of challenge.

These types of individualized clinical judgments are recommended when implementing the auditory memory program described in chapter 8. (See pages 178-193.)

Another issue of implementation concerns the concept of increasing "chunks" versus "number of units." Chunks are defined as related groups of words or components (for example, phrases or related number sequences). The auditory memory program described here, which focuses on sentences only, blends both approaches. Key words are cued by slightly exaggerating volume and intonation. The child is asked to view the speaker's face, a slightly slowed rate of presentation and increased volume are used in the beginning, and natural phrasing is emphasized (for example, by pausing where there are commas and other punctuation marks). The therapist may relate the markers and phrasing to auditory recall (saying, for example, "My voice became louder and higher at the end of that last sentence because it ended in an exclamation point").

This modified "chunking" strategy is recommended in combination with the child's increasing tolerance for length. In the program presented here, sentences and directions become longer and more complicated. Whereas sentences in the beginning involve only single-syllable words, multisyllable words are contained in later sentences. In this way, the therapist can better measure actual progress. This approach also builds the child's tolerance to increasing lengths in very definable terms. Progress is measured by numbers of units or word lengths.

Other memory devices are described. From the beginning, the child becomes vested in his or her own progress by first identifying the specific nature of the problem, identifying how it impacts on academic and social skills, and participating in the solution. The child is asked to describe a good device for recalling information over time. Some children write themselves notes or wear a particular piece of jewelry, while others may wear a watch with an alarm. The point is that the children pinpoint the best strategy for themselves. If that strategy fails, the therapist and child can discuss what happened and perhaps identify another strategy. Regardless of the particular strategy selected, all children should wear watches daily and become accustomed to schedules, time limitations, and appointments as a means of building organizational and anticipatory skills.

In CAPD cases involving severe auditory memory deficits, nonverbal memory skill expansion may need to precede verbal memory focuses. For example, the child may be asked to repeat sequences of sounds involving clapping or musical instruments. This type of activity also is helpful in building an awareness of rhythm, pitch, and rate.

The concept of verbal feedback to oneself is very helpful, especially in cases where auditory memory skills are significantly delayed. This feedback may be spoken aloud (subvocalization) or completed on the thought level (reauditorization). It is particularly helpful in increasing abilities to follow directions. Reauditorization is considered of a higher order than subvocalization. The child may begin with subvocalization techniques and gradually progress to reauditorization. With practice, the process will require less conscious monitoring, and eventually will become automatic.

Other auditory memory techniques include:

- Progressions—Building on previously recalled sequences. Can be used with numbers, letters, unrelated words, or sentences. When sentences are expanded, bring attention to the structural aspects such as subject/predicate, subject/predicate/direct object, and so on. For example:

Kyle

Kyle is

Kyle is a

Kyle is a good

Kyle is a good boy.

- Tape recorders—Lectures are taped at school to review later as often and as slowly as needed.

- Games and expanded stories—

    "I am going grocery shopping and I want to buy an apple."

    "I am going grocery shopping and I want to buy an apple and a banana."

    "I am going grocery shopping and I want to buy an apple and a banana and a coconut . . ."

    The Telephone Game—One child whispers a secret to the next child, who whispers the secret to the next child, and so on.

- Delayed or deferred-recall activities—Skills related to delayed response to directions. Gradually increase the time lag between presentation of directions and response, perhaps beginning with simple directions to be executed after five or ten minutes and gradually progressing to complicated directions to be carried out several hours later. Ask the child what methods of cuing will work best. Suggest a schedule by which the child may recall the direction until the time of completion (for example, "Remind yourself every fifteen minutes until the job is finished. Write yourself a note as a cue"). Strategies that offer organization, predictability, and additional means of cuing seem to work best. When initially presented, the direction may be repeated one time at a slightly slowed and elevated volume, allowing for auditory latency problems (slowed processing time) if necessary.

Incorporate skill integration into auditory memory programs (as well as other CAPD programs). Take every opportunity to incorporate auditory memory skills into other language-learning and language-related skills (speaking, thinking, problem solving, conversations, following directions, taking notes, spelling, reading, and other areas). A good example of this focus is through use of storytelling. Construct a story that contains certain words that have been auditorially identified in advance. Expand the story length, depending on the child's skill levels. Take turns in building the story. Ask the child to "recap" or summarize periodically. The stories may be humorous or realistic. Ask the child to act out the story, write the story, outline the story, alter the ending, change the characters, or discuss its believability. Retell the story and omit certain facts, eliminate the key words, or alter the course of action, and ask the child to identify the changes as they are heard.

On Improving Auditory Discrimination Skills

Tallal (Trace 1993a) stated that individuals with central auditory processing disorder have difficulty integrating temporal information within a 100-millisecond time frame—where many of the temporal acoustic changes fall into speech. Stop consonants and consonant clusters cause more discrimination problems than steady-state signals such as *eh* and *ah*. When the issue of timing arises, a hierarchy of discrimination contrasts becomes apparent. Generally, "longer" signals (phonemes) that have an abundance of acoustic cues are easier to decode or identify than shorter signals. Thus, contrasts that involve numerous acoustic differences should precede those with minimal acoustic differences.

Emphasize *how* contrasted phonemes differ (length, voicing, and so on) in terms the child can understand. Note similarities between phonemes (for example, j and /z/), when appropriate. Effective discrimination probably cannot be taught with only "same or different" exercises.

As therapy progresses, be aware of other "timing" issues. Present contrasts at a slower rate in the beginning of a particular goal, and gradually increase the presentation rate. As with all the therapy focuses, encourage the child to develop both receptive and expressive skills. After a particular contrast is mastered, children enjoy playing "therapist" while you respond.

To identifying phoneme pairs as *same* or *different,* follow this sequencing of materials:

1. High-frequency consonants (for example, /s/ and /f/) versus long vowels

2. High-frequency consonants versus short vowels

3. High-frequency consonants versus low-frequency consonants (for example, /v/ and /l/)

4. Long vowels versus voiced stop consonants (for example, /b/ and /d/)

5. Long vowels versus voiceless stop consonants (for example, /t/ and /k/)

6. Voiced stop consonants versus voiceless stop consonants

7. Long vowels versus consonant clusters (for example, /pr/ and /fr/)

8. Short vowels versus consonant clusters

9. Consonant clusters versus consonant clusters with widely variant acoustic cues (for example, /st/ versus /br/)

10. Consonant clusters versus consonant clusters with somewhat similar acoustic cues (for example, /sh/ versus /st/)

Within the category of short vowel sounds, a significant number of children with CAPD have difficulty with vowel identification and vowel discrimination. In a few cases this may be due to an educational difference; perhaps some of these children were taught reading skills through a sight-vocabulary method rather than a phonic approach. However, in other cases, short-vowel confusion seems more integral to the child's processing problems. Short vowels are "shorter" in duration than their long-vowel counterparts, and thus seem to cause more problems. Remediation of this difficulty should positively affect decoding reading, spelling, and writing skills.

The following sequencing of materials should improve short vowel identification and discrimination:

1. Expose the child to the five short-vowel sounds in isolation on a receptive level.

2. Teach the child to identify various short vowels out of a field of ten. List all five long and short vowels with appropriate identifying marks (for example, ă, ō).

3. Teach the child to identify various short vowels out of a field of only short vowels.

4. Teach the child to identify various combinations of short vowels as "same" or "different."

5. Ask the child to produce each short vowel expressively. (For example, ask, "What is this vowel?")

6. Let the child "play therapist" and complete similar tasks while you act in the student's role. Provide examples of short vowels in various word contexts. Make contrasts between similar words which differ only by the vowel (for example, tap and tape).

Specific materials are provided in chapter 8 that can be used to complement these ideas. Individual programs will reflect individual needs and may involve any combination of focuses and materials provided. The therapy materials reflect reading decoding, speech, speech-reading, and other concerns.

Whenever possible, incorporate a "whole language-like" approach to intervention in which the child is given abundant opportunities to use auditory discrimination skills in a variety of language and language-dependent tasks (for example, following directions, spelling, reading decoding, and writing poetry). In this manner, the child's auditory perception skills also may be strengthened. Additionally, relate auditory discrimination skills to other auditory processing skills such as auditory memory and auditory figure-ground, as needed. For example, ask the child to discriminate between two simple or complex directions, perhaps in the presence of noise.

There is a difference between the auditory discrimination program geared to a child with peripheral hearing impairment and that which is focused on a child with processing disorder. While both populations display difficulties in determining differences between phonemes, some differences exist. Specifically, the basis for such confusions is integral to the poor performance of the ear itself in the former group, while no such problem exists in the latter group. The needs of the group with hearing impairment are somewhat different from those of the group with perceptual impairment in terms of language and communication. The children with hearing impairment are taught to "read" the whole communication set, using all possible available cues. Less emphasis is placed on individual phonemic contrasts. While the children with CAPD also are asked to "read" the entire communication setting, frequently they also are encouraged to fine-tune their discrimination skills in terms of phonemic differences. Such skills are often within a child's "hearing" capabilities and can improve performances in spelling, reading, and following directions as well as other areas.

Although the major focus of intervention in this skill area concerns itself with linguistic contrasts, some children exhibit more fundamental discrimination difficulties in the areas of nonlinguistic stimuli. These children may be unable to distinguish the sound differences between various environmental sounds (for example, a car horn versus a knock on the door). Some children may have difficulties centering on the meaningfulness of the stimuli. Greater difficulties may be experienced with auditory stimuli to which meaning or interpretation have not been attached.

In some cases, the speech-language pathologist must first begin discrimination training with gross environmental sound differences that have clear interpretations attached (such as telephone rings, doorbells, dog barking, and vacuum cleaners). Sounds that differ widely in volume, duration, and frequency are contrasted first, progressing to more subtly varying contrasts that possess less apparent meanings or interpretations. All of these discrimination activities must precede linguistic contrasts when necessary. Individual progress will vary depending on degree of involvement and complicating diagnoses, among other factors. Some children may not progress to higher-order discriminations. (Note that the use of tape recorders to contrast environmental sounds, such as doorbells and dog barking, has limitations. Typical portable tape recorders reduce frequency ranges, thus eliminating some acoustic cues.)

Finally, a brief mention of speech-reading issues is in order. Although the child with CAPD often evidences normal hearing acuity, in reality this child may profit from visual communication cues. This view is consistent with the "whole child" approach to intervention. It also reflects an approach in which auditory discrimination skills are addressed (perhaps at varying points in a therapy program) in a "total communication-like" approach. Specifically, these skills are developed while allowing the child to both "see" and "hear" the contrasted materials.

Therefore, selections for auditory discrimination lessons may reflect speech-reading concerns. These concerns, in terms of phonemic contrasts, may include degree of visibility and whether the contrasts are homophemic (look alike on the lips). Contrasts which look alike (for example, ch/sh, f/v/, p/b/m) rely more heavily on auditory discrimination skills when produced in running speech. The speech-language pathologist may wish to postpone contrasts which involve homophemes until later in therapy. In this way, the child with CAPD and the child with hearing impairment may share similar therapy focuses.

On Improving Auditory Figure-Ground Skills

Auditory figure-ground skills involve an ability to focus on a primary auditory signal in the presence of competing signals (background noise or ambient noise distractions). Auditory figure-ground is also known as *auditory separation* and *auditory selective attention*. Supposedly this skill is largely developed by chronological age six. In reality, this area is frequently a problem in many children who evidence language difficulties. Within this group are a significant number of children with learning disabilities and attention deficit disorder.

Auditory figure-ground deficiencies often have a dramatic impact on classroom performance. Children with this problem may present as one way in quiet, one-to-one settings and appear very different in noisy settings. They may exhibit different behaviors, attitudes, and degrees of attention, depending on the setting. Over time, with repeated frustrating experiences, these children may become behavior problems. They typically do not understand that tolerance to background noise is a problem. Usually, they simply react through distractibility, limited attention, or "tuning out." This is not to imply that all children who "tune out" or who have distractibility problems also have auditory figure-ground problems. However, a significant number of children do. In many of these children, the "symptoms" of the figure-ground deficit may be poor auditory attention, distractibility, and behavioral problems. It is advantageous to look for the possible root cause (that is, auditory figure-ground problems) rather than to focus on eliminating the surface behaviors (distractibility, and so on). Even if the surface behaviors are "controlled," the root cause will remain and probably will surface in other negative behaviors.

Some children also appear to develop a hypersensitivity to noises even when there is little or no background noise. Parents frequently report that their child has begun to turn down the television set and complain about loud speaking levels and odd noises such as the refrigerator sounds. While this is not clearly auditory figure-ground in nature, it sometimes coexists with such problems. Observe how the child reacts to background noise. Does it appear as if all noises become equally weighted (primary and secondary signals blend into one)? This child does not appear to "hear" what has been said. Or does it appear that the child distinguishes between the primary and secondary signals, but under such conditions cannot "remember" what has been said?

When planning programs for auditory figure-ground intervention, several factors must be addressed. Specifically, there are levels of auditory figure-ground challenge that will be categorized in three main levels. The least challenging type of noise, such as that from an air conditioner noise or fan, is considered less difficult to accommodate than noise that is less predictable and nonrepeating. The noises from rain or a clothes dryer are more challenging in that they contain a variety of sounds, but in a fairly repeating pattern. The most challenging noises come from settings in which the noises are constantly changing in frequency and intensity. Typical cafeteria and playground noises fall into this category. Plan the individualized program with regard to increasing tolerance to the specific category of background noise.

Background noises differ in terms of type or category; and intensity levels vary in intragroup as well as intergroup fashions. That is to say, for example, that while the noise levels in any particular cafeteria vary, some cafeterias overall are noisier than others. Therefore, a tolerance to increasing overall intensity must also be planned.

A child does not simply have to learn to tolerate background noises. In real life, the child also must do a variety of tasks in such settings (for example, follow directions, carry on conversations, complete seatwork, follow lecture materials, and other tasks). Therefore, a comprehensive program cannot focus on auditory figure-ground skills exclusively without planning for eventual inclusion of other tasks. The child needs to become proficient at tolerating noises and be able to perform a variety of tasks in a variety of settings.

When other central auditory processing deficits also have been identified, the diagnostic picture becomes more complicated. The most frequent complications are auditory memory for sentences and/or auditory interpretation of directions deficits. Auditory discrimination problems also may appear. Even more challenging is the child who also has transient hearing loss (perhaps due to otitis media) who experiences actual hearing loss on a transient, fluctuating basis.

Examine the entire profile and be sensitive to building tolerances and skill levels from a number of vantage points. For example, build auditory figure-ground skills in isolation; build auditory memory and/or discrimination skills in isolation; then blend the skills in as natural and functional a manner as possible. Regardless of whether taped programs or auditory trainers are used or whether intervention is begun in the therapy office, eventually "therapy" should move out into actual settings such as the school cafeteria and classroom, with the child completing realistic tasks such as taking notes or participating in a group discussion. Skills stand a better chance of being carried over and maintained when the end point in therapy is practical application. When children see that they have the tools to function successfully in a variety of settings and have proof that these tools are useful (for example, better grades, more friends, and other benefits), they are far more likely to maintain and apply them.

Several possible routes can be taken to build auditory figure-ground skills. Commercially produced audiotaped programs and auditory training systems, for example, can be used selectively. In the program presented here, the speech-language pathologist is asked to make audiotapes that become more challenging as skills develop. (See pages 145-146, 179.) Each child will progress at a different rate and have different "complications." Plan individually, and use any combination of strategies at different points to satisfy needs. Whenever possible, encourage the child to work toward functioning as naturally and independently as possible—ideally without instrumentation.

On Improving Auditory Cohesion Skills

For the purposes of this book, the term *auditory cohesion* is used to identify those higher-order auditory processing skills which suggest involvement of cognition, concept development, and elevated linguistic functioning, among other factors. This relatively sophisticated processing skill area may be partially dependent on the development of more fundamental auditory processing skills such as auditory memory and auditory discrimination. This is not to imply that every child who evidences good auditory cohesion skills must necessarily demonstrate good auditory discrimination and memory skills. However, the process of achieving this higher-order level of auditory processing functioning is facilitated by "quality auditory experiences" on which to build language concepts, information, and cognitive skills. "Quality auditory experiences" are those in which communication flows, directions are understood and followed, information is recalled and correlated, and so on.

Since auditory cohesion involves higher-order skills, it would appear that such abilities would serve the child well as the child progresses into the higher grades in school. Academic tasks which require abstraction, inference, analogy, synthesis, summary, categorization, interpretation, and so on, often rely heavily on auditory cohesion skills in both direct and indirect manners. One might say that such skills encourage auditory processing "thinking."

While CAPD populations may demonstrate problems in the auditory cohesion skill area, perhaps the learning disabilities group is the most at risk. When therapy is focused on this skill area, often a positive ripple effect is seen in other aspects of the child's life which require "logic" and problem-solving skills. Therapy focuses for auditory cohesion may include verbal absurdities, analogies, verbal math problems, contingencies, categorizations, decoding of indirect requests, and interpretation of complex directions. This latter task appears to involve more than simple memory of verbally produced information; it also involves the ability to decode how the command must be carried out. When a particular child fails to follow a direction, it may be due not only to a failure to remember what was asked but also a failure to interpret its execution.

Auditory cohesion skills may rely on cortical interhemispheric functioning to some extent. If indeed transcortical communication is involved, there may be inherent sex differences to be noted. Recent research appears to support the notion that the connecting bridge between hemispheres or corpus callosum is larger and shaped differently in females, thus facilitating greater cooperation between parts.

This does not imply that males are more likely to exhibit deficits in all aspects of auditory cohesion as compared to females. It may be, however, that males integrate hemispheric information differently than do females.

Additionally, there may be age implications in terms of skill improvement in the area of auditory cohesion. A question remains as to whether development of this type of hemispheric cooperation is limited by advancing age. These issues are not meant to discourage intervention in this area for any particular individual, but rather to raise awareness of such possible concerns when planning programs.

On Improving Auditory Attention Skills

Auditory attention skills, as used in this book, involve the ability to maintain auditory focus over time even when motivation and interest may be absent. Auditory attention skills appear to be related to several factors including, among other factors, interest, maturation, psychological set, motivation, listening environment, health, attitude, content, auditory memory skills, auditory figure-ground skills, distractions, status of the central nervous system, and hearing. Each child's profile is highly individualized and reflective of these factors. Therefore, it is unlikely that any particular central auditory processing program can be specifically focused on building such skills. Rather, it appears more productive to recognize the various influences on attention and accommodate to them as best as possible on a case-by-case basis.

With academic and social success, many children will demonstrate increased attention. When children see that their listening experiences may be modified and controlled in some ways and that they are thus able to succeed in the classroom, more effort will be put into attending. Attending thus becomes a process that produces positive results. As children receive positive reinforcement for classroom efforts, continued effort is more likely. They must learn to identify the problem as well as the need and take responsibility for their own listening progress. These children must be encouraged to make efforts for their own sense of accomplishment and pride, not simply because they are told to do so under threat of academic failure. A child is more likely to become motivated to attend after being positively reinforced for something done right than after being negatively reinforced after doing something wrong. Catch the child at a time when attention is adequate, and praise the effort.

This approach may be less successful with some children, due to complicating disorders such as attention deficit hyperactivity disorder. The point, however, is that with all children who exhibit attentional limitations, it is advantageous to instill the concept of choices in behavior that result in opportunities for success.

Some "common-sense" techniques may be used to increase attention in terms of time. Children often enjoy the challenge of increasing attention using a minute timer, especially when a reward is possible. In the beginning, expect only a short period of attention, and present simple tasks to be completed within that brief time frame. When a child experiences success from the onset, the child is more likely to want to continue. Remember the interplay of attention, motivation, and self-esteem. Be aware of setting as well. The fewer the visual and auditory distractions, the more likely goals may be achieved. As therapy progresses, lengths of time, settings, and tasks may be changed to reflect increasing skills. Also, investigate rewards that will motivate the child best. (Don't assume that stickers or being line leader will work for all children.) Identify and encourage all aspects of individuality, and give the child a sense of self.

Other strategies, such as preferential seating and focusing on the speaker's face, will help the child maintain attention. In some cases the use of an auditory training system may be recommended for specific settings and tasks. With these systems, the speaker's voice is focused while background noises are abated. In some cases, the classroom may be sound-treated (see page 168). This is a

---

relatively simple and cost-effective process. Kinesthetic cuing, in which the teacher taps the child's shoulder occasionally, also may help the child maintain focus. The teacher also directs frequent questions or comments to the child. The more involved children are in the ongoing discussion or listening task, the more likely they will be to attend.

This area of central auditory processing development is particularly troubling in many children because of its many ripple effects on other areas in the child's life. To varying degrees in many children, overall auditory attention will improve more or less as a by-product of the other factors named above. This area reinforces the notion of treating the whole child rather than simply the central auditory processing disorder.

Auditory Perception

Pamela Gillet, Ph.D. (1993, 51), defines *auditory perception* as "the ability to receive and understand sounds and words." She states that auditory perception is integral to efficient reading skills, conceptual development, and social relationships, among other areas. Various aspects of language learning (including auditory comprehension and receptive vocabulary) may be affected by deficient auditory perception skills. The term *auditory perception* as defined by Gillet has similarities to other terms such as *auditory sound/symbol association* which also have appeared in the literature.

The term *auditory perception* as used in other sources often implies somewhat different meanings. For example, Christine Sloan, Ph.D., defines it as the outcome of auditory processing (Sloan 1991, 1); while Mildred Freburg Berry viewed it as a process which explains how the child's nervous system learns to comprehend and make use of auditory information (Berry 1960, 59).

More simply, in the *Bankson Language Screening Test* (Bankson 1977), the term denotes a part of the test which includes auditory discrimination and auditory memory subtests. Additionally, some Individualized Education Programs (IEPs) identify auditory perception as a major goal area in a general manner and include as subgoals such related focuses as sound blending into words, following of directions, and identification of sounds in the environment.

This book recognizes the reality of these deficits as described by Gillet (1993) in certain children with CAPD, and recommends assessment of auditory perception skills as needed. This may be accomplished formally and informally, directly and indirectly, using the tools for spelling (pages 52-54) and reading (pages 49-51) described in this book, among others.

However, this category of disorder is less prevalent than the five categories of auditory processing identified in chapter 1 (that is, auditory memory, auditory discrimination, auditory figure-ground, auditory cohesion, and auditory attention). Therefore, the speech-language pathologist will need to address auditory perception, and any other central auditory processing disorders, on an individual basis.

Gillet states (1993, 52) that meaning may be attached to auditory symbols of increasing difficulty through the following techniques: repeated presentations until the meaning is internalized; using words in a variety of contexts; limiting vocabulary that is meaningless to the child; and building concepts upon previously acquired information.

Auditory perception as defined above seems to involve a basic problem with abstractions and symbolization. Therefore it is advantageous to initially build the *concept* of a symbol in fundamental form (such as in ordinary play contexts in which a doll symbolizes a baby and a tea set symbolizes actual tableware).

Higher-order symbols may then be introduced, perhaps in the forms of cartoons or holiday symbols (for example, a wreath for Christmas). Sounds in the environment that signal events (passing bells in school, fire alarms, timer bells on the oven, and others) then may be introduced. At that point, the child may be better equipped to associate sounds with symbols as in phonemes and words.

Commercial materials may be helpful to increase the child's sound/symbol associations. Particularly, sections of the *Auditory Discrimination in Depth Program, Revised Edition* (Lindamood and Lindamood 1975) are recommended. Reading approaches that assume a multisensory approach also are advantageous.

This book contains therapy materials that focus on auditory discrimination skills, among other areas. Auditory discrimination is the ability to differentiate sound differences, without attachment of meaning. While materials are provided to improve this skill, additional materials are offered that involve sound/symbol associations and meaning. This represents the logical continuation of skill progression once the child is able to differentiate sound differences. In this way, auditory discrimination skills become blended with auditory perception skills in a functional manner.

Auditory Training, Aural Rehabilitation, and Central Auditory Training

In recent years there has been a move toward a broader, more comprehensive approach to auditory training directed to individuals with hearing impairment. Auditory training is now often viewed as part of a comprehensive program that addresses the overall disabling effect of the hearing impairment on the individual's life (Giolas 1986, 1) rather than on specific skills of sound or word recognition. These programs focus specifically on communication and coping skills. Hearing loss or a hearing impairment of a particular magnitude is differentiated from hearing disability or the effects of that loss upon the individual's everyday life. It is thus recognized that a direct, one-to-one correlation between hearing loss and hearing disability does not exist. Each person's hearing disability will be influenced by a number of factors including, age, motivation, age of onset, and intervention.

Reflecting this change toward broader approaches is the newer concept of *aural rehabilitation,* which incorporates such concerns as psychological adjustment to amplification, speech-reading strategies, language development, and manipulation of the auditory environment. The impact of technology has added to this updated view of aural rehabilitation which now includes the possible use of assistive listening devices, visual communication systems, and tactile information in the reception of signed and/or spoken language. Auditory training thus has become one aspect of aural rehabilitation that focuses on maximizing the use of residual, aided hearing in both comprehending and producing spoken language (O'Brien 1993).

Family members are invited to participate in many such aural rehabilitation programs. Lines of communication are established with appropriate members of the medical community. Individual patients' concerns are addressed both in one-to-one and group contexts. The patient is viewed as a multifaceted individual with a variety of concerns and needs.

In this book, another comprehensive philosophy is applied to the population with CAPD. Communication strategies, management of the environment, psychological factors, and other concerns have been addressed. A comprehensive central auditory training or rehabilitation program is offered here.

Aspects of any comprehensive and multifaceted approach may be influenced by research and experimentation. Possibly the most innovative approach in auditory training in recent years, Auditory Integration Training (also known as Auditory Enhancement Training) has focused largely on those with autism. In *The Sound of a Miracle, A Child's Triumph over Autism* (Stehli 1991), the work of Dr. Guy Berard, a French physician, is described favorably from a parent's perspective. Dr. Berard, a French otolaryngologist, developed innovative auditory training programs for patients with various processing problems including autism, dyslexia, learning disabilities, and attention deficit disorder. He has described his work in *Hearing Equals Behaving* (Berard 1993).

Berard's program involves reducing hyperacuity (or auditory peaks on the audiogram) and developing more normalized hemispheric functioning in terms of processing speech and language. Modified music stimulation is produced, using a device called the Audiokinetron Ears Education and Retraining System (EERS) or Audiokinetron. Among other functions, this system desensitizes hyperacute frequencies through music in which certain frequencies have been filtered out.

Throughout the United States and Canada, there are additional types of integration training in use (for example, Tomatis and Clark).* While the specifics of these programs are still being examined in this country, for the time being some of the fundamental and more broadly accepted concepts may be incorporated into individual programs for persons with CAPD. These concepts may include desensitization in terms of volume and frequency as well as the development of consistent ear preference.

Assistive Listening Devices

Assistive listening devices (ALDs) were first developed to address listening problems of those with hearing impairment. They were never intended to replace hearing aids, but rather to supplement them in particular listening settings. ALDs were designed to transmit sound directly to the ear in an acoustically effective manner.

In recent years, these devices have been used to alleviate some symptoms of central auditory processing disorder. The devices vary in characteristics as well as in price. They range from simple amplifiers to sophisticated infrared systems.

Personal FM (frequency modulated) or infrared systems are devices that improve the signal-to-noise ratio, helping the individual with CAPD to focus on the speaker's voice rather than background noises. Difficulty with ambient noise distractions or background noise is one of the most frequently occurring problems in children with central auditory processing disorder. This skill of focusing on a primary auditory signal while inhibiting irrelevant auditory signals is sometimes known as *selective auditory attention.*

The personal FM system with remote microphone allows the child to move about freely in the classroom. A child with normal peripheral hearing can wear headphones or a neck loop and receiver. The teacher or speaker wears a microphone. This mini-radio system is helpful but not without drawbacks. The batteries of the FM receiver must be regularly recharged and maintained. They also tend to pick up interference from outside sources of radio transmission. The cost is relatively high, and malfunctions can occur frequently.

The infrared system carries sound along infrared light waves and can reduce background noise, improve room acoustics (reverberation common in classrooms), and eliminate distance problems. Similar systems are used with children with hearing impairment. Again, the cost is sometimes prohibitive.

---

*See "Auditory Integration Training" prepared by the American Speech-Language-Hearing Association, Ad Hoc Committee on Auditory Integration and Facilitated Communication, Subcommittee on Auditory Integration Training, David Fabry, Chair; and reported in *Asha,* November 1994, volume 36, pages 55-58. See also S. M. Edelson and L. L. Waddell's undated report, *Auditory Training and Auditory Training Research Project,* published by the Center for the Study of Autism, Newberg, Oregon.

A low-cost assistive listening device was described by Sudler and Flexer (1986). Applications were identified for children with normal hearing who evidenced difficulties with focusing, motivation, and self-regulation. Components of this inexpensive, easy-to-construct, portable system include a small, battery-operated mini-amplifier with input jack and output extension speaker jack with volume control, a tie-clip microphone, and a monaural mini-headset. Sudler and Flexer emphasize that this device should not replace hearing aids or FM systems but may complement them. Applications for children with CAPD attentional difficulties are apparent.

In the past, some children with CAPD have used typical hearing aids. However, because of serious limitations, their usefulness is questionable for the child with normal peripheral hearing. Such hearing aids may amplify auditory signals to uncomfortable levels and intensify background noises as well. New innovations for individuals with hearing impairment include aids that directly connect the aid and the sound source, thus reducing background noise. Another innovation in hearing aids involves digitally programmable aids and integrated circuits. Modifications for individuals with CAPD may be possible in the future.

All types of amplification and listening devices should be evaluated by an audiologist to assure proper fitting and appropriate use. Programs for children with CAPD should always be individually designed, with careful attention paid to both acoustical as well as psychological issues. In reality, some children may find it isolating to wear any device that calls attention to itself.

Individuals with CAPD may be treated through management strategies including use of assistive listening devices or through improvement of the individual's processing skills. In many cases, it may be best to incorporate both approaches. Perhaps the ALD may be viewed as a transition tool, to be used until the child's processing skills can be strengthened. This may not be possible in every case; indefinite reliance on a device may be necessary for some children. Classroom management concerns, including preferential seating, also are critical. Additionally, the student's psychological adjustment to any device is very important. If the child feels stigmatized in any way, the effectiveness of any device becomes questionable.

Therapy Scheduling

Although each case of central auditory processing disorder must be assessed individually, some parameters of scheduling apply generally. Factors such as age of the child, academic placement (for example, self-contained, mainstreamed, inclusion settings), complicating learning problems, attitude, stage of therapy, specific diagnosis, and other concerns must be considered.

Central auditory processing therapy should be viewed as flexible and evolving, with an ultimate goal of varying degrees of independent functioning. Flexibility involves a recognition of possible changes in time needs as well as location needs. Since the ultimate goal is independence, therapy may be scheduled, for example, in the beginning of the year as four half-hour sessions weekly in the therapy room; and by the end of the year may evolve into unscheduled monitoring by the therapist twice monthly within the child's classroom. In many cases, an IEP that allows such flexibility is in the child's best interests.

Therapy for CAPD is unique. Although speech and language dysfunction is addressed in the course of therapy, the basic focus is on the central auditory processing skills that are needed to acquire speech and language more naturally. The speech and language difficulties may be seen as the "symptoms" of the underlying processing disorder. To address the symptoms without first addressing the root bases is simply to sweep the problem under the rug. Some progress may be made in vocabulary acquisition, for example, but more substantial, "natural" gains may be possible once the child has acquired the central auditory processing tools.

Thus, recommendations in terms of time or number of sessions of therapy per week may differ from more traditional approaches. "More" is not necessarily always in the child's best interests, especially when such scheduling involves critical time out of the classroom. Children often feel penalized by time pressures because they must make up classwork they missed while in therapy. This is particularly troublesome because attitude is critical to success in CAPD therapy.

Perhaps therapists should think qualitatively rather than quantitatively in terms of correlating degree of disorder and therapy needs. A program which involves less contact time but allows for frequent, repeated, and varied opportunities for application of skills coupled with adequate monitoring is sometimes most productive.

Pitfalls to Therapy

The following list represents some of the factors that may influence progress in therapy. Several of these issues are more specific to therapy for central auditory processing disorders than to other conditions.

Although these factors do not always limit a favorable prognosis, they should be recognized for the potential impact. Each case is individual, and the therapist should become aware of other potential pitfalls specific to the particular child.

Pitfalls to progress include:

1. An ongoing history of chronic otitis media
2. A loss of hearing sensitivity
3. Age of individual (too old or too young?)
4. Poor attitude
5. Very low self-esteem that severely limits participation and effort
6. Uncontrolled behavior
7. Emotional issues
8. Lack of support from home; poor communication
9. Lack of support from the school or clinical setting; poor communication
10. Inappropriate scheduling
11. Inappropriate academic placement
12. Poor monitoring of carryover skills; failure to plan for transitioning
13. Complicating health issues
14. Poor attendance
15. Poor rapport between the therapist and child
16. Poor rapport between the therapist and team members
17. Failure to plan for long-term needs
18. Complicating language disorders
19. Inappropriate and/or limited diagnosis
20. Failure to recognize specific correlations between various processing disorders and academic performance
21. Failure to recognize the unique relationship between the various processing disorders within an individual profile (for example, how auditory figure-ground difficulties complicate auditory memory problems)
22. Failure to incorporate dynamicism and flexibility into IEP planning.

Other concerns:

Auditory Mirroring

Auditory mirroring is a technique wherein the speech-language pathologist, teacher, or parent repeats all or part of what the child with CAPD has just said. This technique is used in an effort to reduce confusion, to facilitate the flow of conversation, to cue auditory memory skills, or to augment auditory logic skills. Some aspect of what is repeated may be modified, if needed, for clarification or modeling purposes. For example, if it is apparent that the child has "misheard" a particular utterance, the adult may rephrase it appropriately in a modeling manner. For example:

Parent: Please go to the door and see if the mail has come yet.

Child: Why should I go to the store?

Parent: No need to go to the *store*. I said, . . . please go to the *door*. . . . See if the *mail* has come.

Teacher: I had a great winter vacation. My family went skiing in Colorado.

Child: We went skating, too.

Teacher: Oh, you went *skating*? That's terrific. . . Our family did something a little different. We went *skiing*.

Teacher: Name four types of fruit.

Child: Potatoes, corn, and peas.

Teacher: You said, *"Potatoes, . . . corn . . . and peas."* You were able to name *three* types of *vegetables*. Now can you name *four* types of *fruit*?

The mirroring procedure returns the misinformation back to the child in a manner that provides additional auditory and linguistic cues while preserving the child's self-esteem.

Intonation Reading

Intonation, or the pitch, volume, and rate changes in a speaker's verbal expression, conveys meaning to a listener. Teach children with CAPD to tune into these cues when listening to speakers as an additional method of comprehending meaning. *How* an utterance is produced often provides more information than *what* is being said.

Intonation cuing can be practiced both receptively and expressively. Children with CAPDs should be able to "read" the intonation cues produced by others as well as appropriately code their own cues. They also should be aware of the entire communication set as an additional means of comprehension; that is, they should identify and respond to environmental cues such as the particular room setting (classroom, office, and so on), occasion (class discussion, conversation with a friend, and so on), and communication partner (teacher, friend, parent). The child also should respond to facial expressions, body language, and gestures. Each of these factors can alter *how* communication transpires.

Group A

Read the following five sentences aloud. Cue intonation appropriately to the content of each sentence. After each sentence, ask the student which response is most appropriate, and why.

These exercises also may be useful for vocabulary building.

1. I just won the lottery!

    Am I bored, excited, nervous, or ashamed?

2. I don't quite know how to tell you this, but I just had an accident with your new car.

    Am I angry, offended, proud, or embarrassed?

3. The puppy just ran out of the gate into traffic!

    Am I worried, happy, interested, or indifferent?

4. You were supposed to finish your report by this morning. Where is it?

    Am I pleased, annoyed, afraid, or uncertain?

5. You did a terrific job on your room. It's so clean!

    Am I irritated, disappointed, pleased, or impatient?

Group B

Tell the student that the same words can be spoken in different ways and actually mean different things. Ask the student to code his or her own intonation appropriately to the content of the following five sentences. Ask the student why a particular intonation was used.

1. How would you say the following if you were happy? jealous? sarcastic?

    You got an A on your report . . . Great.

2. How would you say the following if you were bored? interested? cooperative?

   You want us to write another ten pages about dinosaurs? Okay.

3. How would you say the following if you were nervous? proud? confident?

   I'm taking my driver's test tomorrow.

4. How would you say the following if you were proud? worried? indifferent?

   I'm having some problems with math lately. I failed my test yesterday.

5. How would you say the following if you were happy? angry? uninterested?

   What do you want for your birthday?

Writing to Dictation

Activities that require the child with CAPD to write to dictation or transcribe what is being said are helpful. These activities are considered to be a prerequisite to note-taking skills. The clinician or teacher may use any grade-level reading materials (paragraph length) to read to the child at a slow rate with full expression and a slightly elevated vocal volume. The child should try to keep pace with the speaker, being more concerned with content or getting the main points than with spelling accuracy. The child should make an effort to maintain auditory attention, keeping eyes on the paper while listening. Afterward, the child should proofread what was written by reading it aloud and listening to his or her own voice cues. The child then should use a highlighting pen to identify the key facts or concepts. These facts or concepts may be placed into a summary or outline.

Note Taking

Note taking is a critical skill that must be learned by junior high school. It is a challenging task for children with CAPD because it involves several higher-order linguistic functions that must be used rapidly. The student must "hear" the lecture material, recall it accurately while repeating it mentally, summarize it, and then write it down in some organized, decodable manner. All of this transpires while additional lecture material is being produced. Since it is suspected that timing issues are relevant to processing difficulties in some children with CAPD, and because many of these children have other language impairments (for example, expressive language, receptive vocabulary, spelling difficulties), this process becomes all the more difficult. Some children have auditory-visual integration problems; that is, difficulty with blending information from the ears and eyes simultaneously. If the materials are presented in settings with background noise, children with figure-ground difficulties are even more challenged.

Note-taking skills rely on higher-order processing skills and may be placed within the category of Auditory Cohesion. The form on page 162 may be used to develop these skills gradually. Encourage the child to act on any particular skill in more than one way. For example, teach the child not only to recall lecture materials and summarize them in an orderly fashion, but also to put the notes into paragraph form (as in report writing), and then present them orally (as in oral reporting). Growth and stability are encouraged whenever language skills can be manipulated and revamped into related formats.

Develop note-taking skill gradually, with both context and task increasing over time. At first, practice in the therapy room, without auditory distractions and with materials limited to three or four sentences. Stand close to the student, and present the material at a slow-normal rate. Help the child identify the key words to be transcribed—those which provide the heart of the material. Discourage the child from wasting valuable time on incidental words such as articles, and help the child to learn to transcribe in a telegraphic fashion. Teach the child to identify key words by how they are coded by the speaker. Often these words are produced at a slightly slower rate and louder level as they are emphasized by the speaker. Teach the student to listen to *how* speech is produced as well as to *what* is being said.

Examine the transcribed notes, and ask the student to explain what the notes mean and why they are important. Make alternate suggestions for coding more efficiently. Explain and reinforce the strategy of *reauditorization* (recalling within the mind of materials heard previously). Teach the child to use this strategy in order to reproduce the information in summarized or edited form.

When the child is able to effectively take notes, increase the challenge level. Over time, encourage the child to take notes from different speakers (each speaking at different rates with varying styles), in different settings (classrooms with varying noise levels), and for longer periods of time. Elevate the level of materials, and present more abstract or technical information. Base these decisions on the child's individual capabilities and needs.

Note-Taking Form

Use this form to practice transcribing key facts in decodable form. Then compile the facts into paragraph form. Finally, proofread your paragraph by reading it aloud.

Taking Notes

Key Facts

1. _____
   _____

2. _____
   _____

3. _____
   _____

4. _____
   _____

5. _____
   _____

6. _____
   _____

7. _____
   _____

8. _____
   _____

Summary

_____
_____
_____
_____
_____

Proofreading

Proofreading is another strategy that is essential to writing tasks. Whenever possible, encourage students to proofread or check their own written materials for technical errors (spelling, grammar, and so on) as well as communicability (Does this say something in an understandable form?). Students may not be able to rely solely on reauditorization strategies to complete this task. Therefore, encourage them to use another strategy called *subvocalization*. This strategy involves actually repeating the materials aloud, as opposed to saying them in one's mind. Subvocalization can be done very discreetly with minimal volume. The advantage of this type of self-cuing is that the student is again encouraged to use *how* the material sounds as a means of identifying grammatical markers (that is, pauses may cue commas and periods, increased pitch and volume may cue exclamation points, and so on). Students with CAPD often speak better then they write. When asked, "Does this sound right to you?" or "Does it sound like you would actually say it?" these students are likely to respond in the negative and subsequently make the appropriate revisions in their writing. Teach the students to look at words and ask themselves, "Does this look right?"

Syllabication cues may also be used in proofreading. When students encounter difficult-to-spell words, they may use the numbers of syllables "heard" as a word-attack strategy. Encourage the child to identify which syllable is accented by asking, "Which syllable is longer, louder, and higher-pitched than the others?" Polysyllabic words broken down in this fashion often become more manageable to decode and spell.

Proofreading Exercise

The paragraph on page 164 contains many errors. Have the students use it to practice auditory proofreading techniques.

Ask them to create a second paragraph to complete the story and use proofreading techniques to check that paragraph, too.

Proofreading Exercise

It were a cold and snowing mourning! When I looked out my windo, I see glistened trees and drifting rain. I quick turn the radio on to heared if my school was closing. After listened to a long list, I finally heared my school name. Its closed for the day? I run to waked up my lttl sistre and telled her the grate news. Exsited, we got dress too go sledding so fast. But, frist we had too ate breckfast.

_____

_____

_____

_____

_____

_____

_____

_____

_____

_____

_____

Progress in Therapy: Case Studies

Michael

Michael is the 11-year-old, sixth-grade boy described in chapter 1 (see page 18). He was classified as learning disabled and attended resource room daily. Reading comprehension and language skills were reported by his mother as weak. Michael's mother indicated that focusing, following directions, and applying logic also caused problems for Michael. He had generally poor peer relationships and suffered from low self-esteem.

Central auditory processing testing indicated problems with auditory figure-ground, auditory memory for sentences, auditory interpretation of directions, and auditory cohesion. Deficits in delayed recall as well as receptive and expressive vocabularies also were noted. Michael was opposed to use of an auditory trainer, fearing that other children would make fun of him. Use of one therefore was not considered a therapy option.

Michael began therapy begrudgingly. Although he was basically friendly and cooperative, he seemed to resent "more" testing and therapy. He expressed feelings of frustration in terms of school performance and social relationships. The most important aspect of therapy at that early point was to empower Michael—to demonstrate to him the exact nature of his listening difficulties and discuss possible strategies for intervention. Assuring him that he was not alone in these types of problems seemed to help, as did pointing out that his difficulties did not indicate low intelligence. Michael completed the "talents" chart (Identify and Develop Your Talents, page 119) and was pleasantly surprised by how many areas he excelled in without realizing it. He was then given the Self-Affirmations chart (see page 120) and told that just as football team players need to be "psyched" before a game, so must he. He was asked to choose a daily affirmation carefully, based on reality as he saw it.

The first session was spent in mapping out the focus of Michael's program and detailing his responsibilities. He was led to understand that without his active input and participation, improvements would be unlikely. An agreement was made among Michael, the therapist, and Michael's mother to share responsibilities toward a common goal.

Michael was given weekly assignments that were progressively challenging. He was asked to chart progress and problems daily. At the beginning of each session, he and the therapist discussed problems and problem-solving strategies. He was asked to maintain schedules and homework and appointment charts, organize his desk and room, and complete regular chores at home.

Michael became involved in his program, and this awareness and confidence produced positive effects in both the classroom and in his social life. He progressively became more alert to listening settings that were causing problems (for example, noisy classrooms) and was vigilant about applying strategies. As he saw the positive results, he became more and more vested in the process. He felt better about himself because he took pride in his better grades in school, and he enjoyed the positive reinforcement from others. He became an "active participant" and not just a "case" because he saw value in the program. He was not there simply because he was told to go to therapy. He viewed the therapist and himself as team members.

Other aspects of Michael's central auditory processing profile also were addressed. An increasing auditory memory for sentences was followed by an increasing ability to carry out directions. This in turn was followed by an increasing ability to carry out directions (both immediate and delayed) in noise. The memory/figure-ground program contained here (see pages 178-192) was used.

After four weeks of the program, auditory cohesion deficits began to be addressed and progressively challenged. Michael's basic interest in learning and fundamental intelligence accelerated this process. He showed interest in the "logic" of responses and enjoyed trying to "fool" the therapist with auditory exercises such as riddles, contingencies, and absurdities. (See chapter 8 for examples.)

After three months of therapy (one hour weekly), auditory memory, cohesion, and figure-ground skills were retested and found to be greatly improved. Some improvements were noted in vocabulary skills. Michael was provided with a transition program (see chapter 9), for purposes of integrating into a school-based program which would address the remaining vocabulary and auditory cohesion deficits and monitor ongoing memory and figure-ground skills. Periodic retesting was recommended. Michael understood that continued skills must be actively maintained and that the process was a complicated, ongoing one involving psychological, therapeutic, and academic factors.

Lori

Lori is the seven-year-old girl described in chapter 1 (see page 20). Testing had indicated moderate to severe difficulties in all five skill areas of central auditory processing. Lori also exhibited attention deficit hyperactivity disorder.

Lori's home life, although apparently loving and supportive, appeared disorganized and a bit frantic in pace. Homework assignments were not completed, appointments were canceled without notice, arrival for appointments was often late, and so on.

Although the approach to therapy was explained to the mother in terms of strategies to be used at home, coordination with the teacher, maintenance of chore lists, and other factors, it didn't appear that the information was well understood. The parent seemed to view therapy as something she brought her child to each week that did not have any additional responsibilities throughout the week. Although Lori was a personable, energetic child, these conditions severely hampered progress. The hyperactivity component to her diagnostic profile complicated matters even further. For such a child, organization, scheduling, carryover strategies, and other cues for focus and attention were considered extremely important.

After these patterns were observed over a period of several weeks, the parent was again counseled regarding therapy focuses and approaches. The need for a joint-effort approach was emphasized. The mother agreed that this was important, but mentioned difficulties with so many responsibilities, scheduling, and so on. She blamed Lori's school for mishandling her, and she maintained that it was the school's responsibility to remediate Lori's "behavior problems." The mother canceled the following appointment, stating that she had a change in work schedule and would call the following week about a new appointment period. She never called back. Lori was not seen for therapy after that point.

In this case, unless the pattern could be modified, therapy progress would continue to be minimal or nonexistent. Discharge from therapy under such circumstances is a viable alternative. Perhaps a "temporary" discharge could be arranged so the door could remain open to trying again later.

Quantitative versus Qualitative Issues

Progress in individual cases often may be viewed in terms of quantitative versus qualitative issues. Perhaps children whose diagnostic profiles suggest quantitative differences in CAP function (that is, whose profiles mimic the characteristics of a younger child or demonstrate "less" of something) appear to "catch up" in some ways. Those children whose profiles suggest qualitative involvement (that is, do not mimic the characteristics of a younger child and are more "disordered" may never "catch up" and may require individualized strategies or mechanisms to cope.

Classroom Acoustical Considerations

Because children with central auditory processing disorder frequently experience difficulty in a typical classroom setting, Hart (1983) and others have suggested a number of acoustical modifications. The fundamental concern is to create a listening environment that facilitates attention without distraction from competing, irrelevant noises. The classroom should "enhance the clarity and intensity of informational messages from the teacher and other students" (Hart 1983, 344).

Specific standards are provided by Hart as adapted from Ross (1978) and Borrild (1978). The following listing represents a further adaptation which reflects classroom accommodations that are practical in terms of cost and effort. These alterations may be implemented in conjunction with preferential seating. Most cases will not require many of these alterations.

1. Signal-to-noise ratio—This ratio should be at least +10 decibels difference (that is, the teacher's voice should be at least 10 decibels louder than ambient noises). This may be accomplished through instrumentation (that is, use of an auditory trainer) and by speaking a little louder.

2. Distance between speaker and listener—A distance of 6 to 8 feet is considered optimal in terms of clarity and volume of speech.

3. Sound transmission—Completely seal all intersections of the wall to floor, ceiling, and other openings such as those to windows and corridors.

4. Classroom configurations and size—In order to create a diffuse sound field, classrooms that approximate a square shape are preferable. Dimensions of 25 feet by 30 feet with 12-foot-high ceilings are considered optimal in regular classrooms.

5. Design recommendations—The classroom may contain three main areas— a large central area for group interaction and two smaller areas along end walls for individual and small-group activities. Place the small-group areas under a 7-foot-high, sound-absorbent ceiling and soffit. Also cover the end wall with sound absorbers.

6. Flooring—Cover the entire floor area with carpeting to absorb and muffle sounds at their source.

7. Hallway noise reduction—Seal the entry door with vinyl or felt sound stripping. Carpet the hallway floors, and fit the ceilings with acoustical tiles.

8. Wall attenuation—Seal all cracks, construct double walls, install fiberglass sound insulation, drop ceilings as needed, and install heavy draperies and acoustic tiles.

9. Lighting—Build fluorescent lighting fixtures into the ceiling, making certain the light is not too harsh. Install task lights in the small-group work areas.

10. Chalkboards—Chalkboards provide efficient reflective surfaces for sound transmission that maximize the teacher's voice. The longer the board, the better in terms of reinforcing the teacher's voice as well as allowing lateral mobility.

Goals for Individualized Education Programs

The following list contains representative short-term goals for the five skill areas of central auditory processing dysfunction. Examples of strategies follow the list. Examples of computerized IEP goals also are provided.

Because individual diagnostic profiles are so specific to each child, some types of computerized Individualized Education Programs (IEPs) may not be acceptable. However, specific formats may be used repeatedly and individualized easily.

Additional goals of a related nature (reading, spelling, proofreading, organizational skills, and do on) also may be included in a complete IEP.

- -

Sample Short-Term Goals

For Auditory Memory

1. The child will increase auditory memory skills for sequenced numbers from _____ (number) units to _____ (number) units by _____ (date).

2. The child will increase auditory memory skills for sequenced words from _____ (number) units to _____ (number) units by _____ (date).

3. The child will increase auditory memory skills for sentences from _____ (number) words to _____ (number) words by _____ (date).

4. The child will be able to immediately carry out _____ (number) simple, one-step commands with _____% accuracy by _____ (date).

5. The child will be able to immediately carry out _____ (number) complex, two-step commands with _____% accuracy by _____ (date).

6. The child will be able to delay execution of _____ (number) simple, one-step commands for _____ (time) with _____% accuracy by _____ (date).

For Auditory Figure-Ground

1. The child will improve auditory figure-ground skills as evidenced by the ability to correctly execute one-step (or two-step) commands in the presence of ambient noise (identify type) with _____% accuracy out of a field of _____ (number) by _____ (date).

2. The child will be able to complete a directed, complex motor task (for example, cleaning out a desk or categorizing books) in the presence of ambient noise (identify type) within a time-frame of _____ minutes by _____ (date).

Copyright © 1995 by Communication Skill Builders, a division of The Psychological Corporation / All rights reserved / 1-800-228-0752
Central Auditory Processing Disorder / Dorothy A. Kelly, D.A. / ISBN 0761631623

For Auditory Cohesion

1. The child will be able to respond appropriately to contingency requests (for example, "If ____, then ____") with ____% accuracy out of a field of ____ (number) by ____ (date).

2. The child will be able to correctly respond to simple riddles with ____% accuracy out of a field of ____ (number) by ____ (date).

3. The child will be able to reproduce in reverse order a sequence of ____ (number) digits by ____ (date).

4. The child will be able to correctly identify a category heading (for example, cars) when presented with five examples of members (for example, Chevrolet, Buick, Ford, Dodge, Toyota) with ____% accuracy in ____ (number) trials.

5. The child will be able to delay execution of ____ (number) complex, two-step commands for ____ (time) with ____% accuracy by ____ (date).

For Auditory Discrimination

1. The child will improve auditory discrimination skills for word pairs differing by a single phoneme in the ____ (initial, medial, final) position for ____ (number) out of a field of ____ (number) to ____ (number) out of a field of ____ (number) by ____ (date).

2. The child will improve auditory discrimination skills for similar phrases differing by a single word from ____ (number) out of a field of ____ (number) to ____ (number) out a field of ____ (number) by ____ (date).

3. The child will improve auditory discrimination skills for similar sentences differing by a single word from ____ (number) out of a field of ____ (number) to ____ (number) out of a field of ____ (number) by ____ (date).

4. The child will be able to correctly identify single consonant (or vowel) phonemes when presented with a written listing as produced by the therapist with ____% accuracy when presented within a field of ____ (number) by ____ (date).

5. The child will improve auditory discrimination for single phoneme contrasts (for example, C/C, C/V, V/V) when presented by the therapist and identify pairs as *same* or *different* with ____% accuracy within a field of ____ (number) by ____ (date).

Central Auditory Processing Disorder / Dorothy A. Kelly, D.A. / ISBN 0761631623

For Auditory Attention

1. The child will be able to maintain auditory focus for _____ (number) minutes for the purpose of taking notes in a distraction-free environment by _____ (date).

2. The child will be able to maintain auditory focus for _____ (number) minutes for the purpose of taking notes in the presence of auditory (or auditory/visual) distractions by _____ (date).

3. The child will be able to maintain auditory focus for _____ (number) minutes for the purpose of listening to a class lecture as evidenced by sitting attentively by _____ (date).

Strategies

Some suggested strategies are identified below. Such strategies may be noted on procedural sections of IEPs.

subvocalization	reduced rate of production
reauditorization	increased volume
chunking	modifying listening environment
reauditorized or subvocalized proofreading	preferential seating
	mirroring
exaggerated intonation	visual imagery

Computerized Individualized Education Programs

Computerized IEPs may be organized with overhead goals and supportive goals (or otherwise noted terms) in a format such as that shown on pages 172-173. Numerical codes identify both overhead and supportive goals.

These goals are more general than the examples provided above, and they do not identify strategies or procedures. There is a trend toward presenting these types of plans. As long as the listing of possible goals (and related goals) within the computer index is appropriate and extensive, these plans may be functional.

A separate group of goals is provided for tasks involving directions. Skills related to the following of directions are different from those related to auditory memory (for example, many children can recall sentence sequences and cannot carry out a direction).

The following list is representative only and should be expanded considerably.

Sample Computerized Individualized Education Programs

1. _____ will improve auditory memory skills.

   a. _____ will repeat a sequence of 4 or 5 numbers.

   b. _____ will repeat a sequence of 2 or 3 unrelated words.

   c. _____ will repeat a sequence of 6 words in sentence form.

   d. _____ will be able to restate oral directions involving one step.

   e. _____ will be able to restate oral directions involving two steps.

2. _____ will improve auditory discrimination skills.

   a. _____ will identify two-word combinations which may differ by a single phoneme as *same* or *different*.

   b. _____ will be able to identify two-word combinations that may differ by a single short vowel sound as *same* or *different*.

   c. _____ will be able to repeat sentences verbatim that differ by a single word.

   d. _____ will identify specific sentences spoken by the therapist among a choice of three similar sentences in written form.

   e. _____ will identify specific short vowel phonemes when produced by the therapist.

3. _____ will improve auditory figure-ground skills.

   a. _____ will be able to follow a one-step command in the presence of cafeteria-like background noise.

   b. _____ will be able to maintain a conversation for five minutes in the presence of air conditioner-like background noise.

   c. _____ will be able to ask two questions in the presence of low-volume cafeteria-like background noise.

   d. _____ will be able to talk on the telephone for three minutes in the presence of air conditioner-like noise.

   e. _____ will be able to carry out a two-step command in the presence of typical classroom noise.

(continued)

Sample Computerized Individualized
Education Programs (continued)

4. _____ will improve auditory cohesion skills.

   a. _____ will be able to identify the nonsensical portion of a sentence when orally presented.

   b. _____ will be able to correctly respond to riddles when orally presented.

   c. _____ will correctly complete analogies when orally presented.

   d. _____ will correctly respond to "logic" questions when orally presented.

   e. _____ will correctly identify the process needed to solve verbal math problems when orally presented.

5. _____ will improve auditory attention skills.

   a. _____ will be able to maintain focus for five minutes during a lectured activity.

   b. _____ will be able to maintain auditory attention for ten minutes of conversation.

   c. _____ will be able to maintain attention for one-half hour during a group activity.

   d. _____ will be able to identify key words when heard during the reading of an excerpt from a social studies textbook.

   e. _____ will be able to maintain attention during a five-minute telephone conversation.

6. _____ will be able to follow directions.

   a. _____ will be able to follow a one-step command immediately.

   b. _____ will be able to follow a two-step command immediately.

   c. _____ will be able to carry out a one-step command after one hour.

   d. _____ will be able to carry out a two-step command when presented in noise after two hours.

   e. _____ will be able to carry out a three-step command after two days.

Therapy Log for
Central Auditory Processing Intervention

Child's Name:	Grade/Placement:

Specific Diagnosis:

Speech-Language Pathologist:

Date:

Date:

Date:

Date:

Date:

Date:

Date:

Date:

Date:

General Order of Therapy Focuses

All cases of central auditory processing disorder present highly individualized profiles. Therapy intervention cannot be approached in a homogeneous or "cookie cutter" manner. An individual case may involve a combination of difficulties which impact uniquely on one another and on language-dependent activities.

The following sequence suggests a general order that may be used in cases in which all of the major skill areas are affected. This order should be adapted on an as-needed basis. For example, if auditory memory is affected, but only very mildly so, and auditory discrimination appears more severely affected, the speech-language pathologist may consider working on the latter area initially. This sequence also suggests a type of hierarchy of challenge; that is, auditory memory appears to be a lower-order skill area than auditory cohesion, which may rely in part on auditory memory to actualize. Auditory attention is considered a separate skill area but can be developed throughout any particular program.

Order of Intervention:

1. Auditory Memory

2. Auditory Discrimination

3. Auditory Figure-Ground

4. Auditory Cohesion

Skills are synergistic in nature, impacting on one another in numerous ways. For example, a child with an auditory memory problem as well as an auditory figure-ground problem may demonstrate poorer auditory memory problems in the classroom than in the therapy room. Similarly, a child may be able to recall sequences of words in sentence form immediately, yet be unable to act upon a direction either immediately or later.

For these reasons and others, each child's program must be individualized. Select materials for particular children very carefully. Make choices after an in-depth analysis of assessment results and after consultations with parents, classroom teachers, and other informants.

8

Therapy Materials

Overview

This chapter contains specific strategies and techniques for four of the five main skill areas (auditory memory and following directions, auditory figure-ground, auditory discrimination, and auditory cohesion).

Because overall auditory attention may be contingent on several factors, including interest, modification of the listening environment, and development of the various skill areas, here it is not treated in the same manner as the other four skill areas. Strategies for encouraging stronger attentional or focusing skills are listed in summary form (see page 233).

Therapy materials are provided for each of the four skill areas. The chapter has been divided into three sections which reflect these focuses.

- Section 1 focuses on building an auditory memory for sentences first, then progresses to following of directions (immediate and delayed), and then to following directions (immediate and delayed) with ambient noise distractions.

- Section 2 deals with auditory discrimination and emphasizes typical problematic contrasts (for example, stop consonants and consonant blends).

- Section 3 focuses on auditory cohesion development and emphasizes a variety of higher-order auditory tasks.

Each lesson contains a "turnaround" activity in which the child must manipulate the information in some expressive form. This process is considered important because it requires application, carryover, and concept understanding.

The sections may be used as needed—not necessarily in entirety. Specific directions are given for each section. All exercises can be carried out within the therapy room, classroom, or home with minimal accommodation.

Section 1:
Auditory Memory and Following Directions

Children with CAPD often have difficulties applying auditory memory skills in practical action form (following directions). These children also commonly display greater difficulties in noisy settings. These problems are addressed in Section 1.

Section 1 has been divided into five subsections:

    1A: Auditory Memory—Recall of Lengthening Units

    1B: Following Directions—Immediate Response

    1C: Following Directions—Delayed Response

    1D: Following Directions in Noise—Immediate Response

    1E: Following Directions in Noise—Delayed Response

Section 1D requires a therapist-made audiotape of white noise (for example, air conditioner or fan noise). Section 1E requires a more challenging therapist-made audiotape of complex noise (for example, conversations or cafeteria or playground noises).

Directions for Section 1

Section 1A:
Auditory Memory—Recall of Lengthening Units

Section 1A contains a total of 90 sentences, grouped in tens, ranging from four to 12 units/words in length.

The purpose of this section is to build auditory memory, using sentences with only one syllable. Students are not required to complete directions. The ability to follow directions requires more sophisticated functioning than the simple recall of sentences. Section 1A is designed to build solid auditory memory skills that can provide a foundation for subsequent higher-order processing tasks.

Initiate one level below current performance level. For example, if the student's auditory memory has been identified as limited to five unit/word lengths, begin the program at the four-unit/word level. This policy will provide the student with early success and an impetus to continue.

Skill levels are noted in terms of numbers of units/words. For example, the student may be able to recall 10 units/words with 50% accuracy in two trials. This means that the student can accurately recall 10 units/words half the time or, in this example, during one trial. Students may continue practicing with any given task until 90% to 100% accuracy is achieved on two or more successive trials.

If the student has not achieved the goal after adequate effort has been made, discontinue the task. Document performance, using the Task Accuracy Form (page 193).

Section 1B:
Following Directions—Immediate Response

Section 1B also has 90 sentences, grouped in tens, ranging from four to 12 unit/ words in length. These sentences require the student to complete an action. All the sentences contain single-syllable words so that progress and status can be clearly specified. All tasks are to be completed within the immediate environment and within the immediate time frame. Materials needed to complete these tasks are commonly available.

This part of the program is considered more challenging than Section 1A in that the student is now being asked to apply memory skills to specific tasks.

Initiate this part of the program at one level below performance level, and progress to age-appropriate expectation levels whenever possible.

Section 1C:
Following Directions—Delayed Response

Section 1C contains 45 sentences, grouped in fives, ranging from four to 12 words in length. This part of the program is considered more challenging than Sections 1A and 1B, in that it contains one- and two-syllable words and requires deferred action. The sentences may be accessed by audiotape or by having a clinician, teacher, or parent read them aloud to the student.

Various techniques or strategies may help the student to retain the required command until the specified time of completion. For example, if the student is asked to complete a task "after dinner" (which is perhaps six hours away), encourage the student to use the techniques of subvocalization or reauditorization as often as needed. See "On Improving Auditory Memory Skills" (pages 139-141) for more strategies.

Section 1D:
Following Directions in Noise—Immediate Response

Section 1D of this program contains 45 sentences, grouped in fives and composed of one-, two-, and three-syllable words. An immediate response is required for each sentence presented with background noise.

The noise present in Section 1D is the type which is considered less distracting and less challenging than the noise used in Section 1E. Specifically, white noise (air conditioner or fan noise) may be used in Section 1D, and more complex noise (cafeteria or playground noise) may be used in Section 1E. Make simple audiotapes of various noises of increasing levels of challenge, and modify Sections 1D and 1E as needed for the individual student. (For example, increase the volume.)

It is important that the student learn to deal with noise in a functional manner. The student should not only be able to tolerate it during common, self-directed activities, but also should be able to follow directions, participate in conversations, and generally maintain auditory focus and attention.

In Sections 1D and E, encourage students to actively participate in the process of screening out noise distractions. Help them to realize that this process involves responsibility and consistent effort on their part.

If the student has considerable difficulty with either Section 1D or 1E of the program, modify the procedure slightly. While reading the sentences aloud to the student, lower the volume of background noise. Use a slightly louder and exaggerated tone of voice and natural gestures.

Section 1E:
Following Directions in Noise—Delayed Response

Section 1E also contains 45 sentences of one-, two-, and three-syllable words. The sentences, grouped in fives and presented with more challenging background noise (cafeteria noise or conversation noise), require delayed responses.

This part of the program presents the most difficult tasks. Students must respond to increasingly complex commands in a deferred manner. If needed, modify the presentation as noted in Section 1D.

Four-unit\word lengths

1. I shut the door.
2. We like to sing.
3. The dog is brown.
4. There are five birds.
5. The man is short.
6. The phone rings twice.
7. The drink is sweet.
8. They all ate well.
9. The floor is wet.
10. Bill has been gone.

Five-unit\word lengths

1. The dog has a leash.
2. The man takes a pill.
3. The drink is very tart.
4. Tim's car has four wheels.
5. We want the house cleaned.
6. Jill is a tall girl.
7. We go to the store.
8. I am good at math.
9. You are a thin boy.
10. That is a green frog.

Six-unit\word lengths

1. The man played a loud song.
2. The cows graze in the field.
3. We will go for a walk.
4. The old man took his pill.
5. The food is on the way.
6. I like to watch the show.
7. The old horse walks so slow.
8. Pat and Joe are good friends.
9. He took me to the house.
10. We rode in a fast car.

Seven-unit\word lengths

1. The rat ran from the black cat.
2. My new car is black and white.
3. The glass on the floor is cracked.
4. She is a fine friend of mine.
5. We all know how that stove works.
6. Steve likes to paint with his brush.
7. Joan tied the rope to the tree.
8. A saw is used to cut wood.
9. The bird flew down from the branch.
10. A mouse is so hard to catch.

Eight-unit\word lengths

1. The hot sun on our backs feels good.
2. I will call my friend on the phone.
3. My house is on a street called Elm.
4. The boy is too young to play ball.
5. I like to eat fruit and drink milk.
6. My mom does not like to drink juice.
7. The bright sun lit up the dark field.
8. Jack made a tape of Jim's first class.
9. I read my long script to the class.
10. The squash patch grew in the spring months.

Nine-unit\word lengths

1. You and I like to swim at the beach.
2. I will swim and play ball at the pool.
3. My young aunt has blue eyes and blond hair.
4. We read books on birds and dogs all year.
5. When we are at the store, we buy food.
6. A cold drink would feel good down my throat.
7. Bill used a leash to keep his dog safe.
8. A horse will buck if it is not tame.
9. Card tricks are fun to show to your friends.
10. The path from here to my house is long.

10-unit\word lengths

1. A man with a blue shirt works in the store.
2. The flag on the pole is red, white, and blue.
3. I like to swim when I am in the pool.
4. In school I like to read books and write songs.
5. My brand-new shirt is black, green, and bright pink.
6. The car came to a stop at the stop sign.
7. The first ray of sun shone on the cool swamp.
8. Jon took ten dimes for the work he had done.
9. There was more than one game for Kim to choose.
10. A day at the splash park is fun and wet.

11-word\unit lengths

1. The sheet on the bed is light green and dark red.
2. Next week I will fix the phone that does not ring.
3. I will not wear the blouse with blue stripes on it.
4. When my friends and I play, we play in the park.
5. I don't know if we should call Aunt Joan next week.
6. I love to feed the ducks on the coast of Maine.
7. My leg will heal if my cast stays on for months.
8. To drive a car, you must first pass a hard test.
9. The light will not work if the bulb is not new.
10. My hands are so cold from the snow on the ground.

12-word/unit lengths

1. We left the new lamp on in the house late last night.
2. I went to the pool and had fun with my good friends.
3. Bob likes to run in gym with his friends who train hard.
4. She likes to go to the store on the street near us.
5. When Jill talks to her friends, she makes them laugh out loud.
6. This week I have to go to the bank and the store.
7. My friend and I must go to the store to buy books.
8. The small fish swam out to the big sea to find food.
9. My friend Ben is not good in math or gym these days.
10. The girl has brown hair, blue eyes, and teeth that are straight.

Section 1B:
Following Directions—Immediate Response

Four-unit\word lengths

1. Draw a red box.
2. Touch your right ear.
3. Bend at the waist.
4. Sit on a chair.
5. Stand on your toes.
6. Look out the door.
7. Brush your hair back.
8. Lift your pen high.
9. Show me your teeth.
10. Turn to your left.

Five-unit\word lengths

1. Hop on your left foot.
2. Draw a big blue bird.
3. Box three small brown fish.
4. Take off your right shoe.
5. Look at the blue bird.
6. Tap your right knee once.
7. Find two small, red things.
8. Pick up one black pen.
9. Clap your hands three times.
10. Count to 12, then 10.

Six-unit\word lengths

1. Write your first name two times.
2. Think of four ways to play.
3. Bend your right hand back twice.
4. Turn a page of a book.
5. Shake your head, then smile twice.
6. Read four words from a book.
7. Draw a red bird with wings.
8. Count to five once out loud.
9. Draw a check in a star.
10. Tap your cheek, then your foot.

Seven-unit\word lengths

1. Drop a black pen on the desk.
2. Draw a blue line through a box.
3. Look at the floor, then the door.
4. Jump up four times, then blink once.
5. Write the word *book* on this page.
6. Pick up a book, then drop it.
7. Shade your eyes with both your hands.
8. Cup your ears with both your hands.
9. Smile while you clap your hands once.
10. Close your mouth, then touch your head.

Eight-unit\word lengths

1. Draw a red line next to a box.
2. Find two black or blue pens with caps.
3. Rub your left knee with your right hand.
4. Close your eyes while you touch your nose.
5. Write your last name, then your first name.
6. Touch your ear and nose with your hand.
7. Stretch your right arm high in the air.
8. Wink with your left eye while you cough.
9. Touch your hair and chin with your thumb.
10. Draw three brown lines next to a tree.

Nine-unit\word lengths

1. Spell your last name and then your first name.
2. Ask if you can go to the store now.
3. Turn to your left and then to your right.
4. Trace the shape of a heart and a star.
5. Mark this page with five lines at the top.
6. Use your hand to show how tall you are.
7. Tell the names of your mom and your dad.
8. Hide a pen in a high place near you.
9. Move your chair to a spot near the door.
10. Fold this page in two parts, then in four.

10-unit\word lengths

1. Show me what you can draw in a small box.

2. Sing or hum a song that makes you feel glad.

3. Go to the door, then go to the far wall.

4. Hold your left arm tightly with your right hand.

5. Place a pen and a dime on a high shelf.

6. Kick the leg of the big chair near the door.

7. Sit on the desk, then sit on your own chair.

8. Stand up, then sit down, then blink your eyes twice.

9. Jump up three times and then clap your hands once.

10. Name two or three foods that taste sweet and cold.

11-unit\word lengths

1. Count from 1 to 6, and then from 8 to 12.

2. Name five tools to clean a house or fix a car.

3. Find two things in the room that are black and white.

4. Tell why girls and boys like to play games at school.

5. Tell what times you go to sleep, eat lunch, and play.

6. Name two boys' and three girls' names that start with R.

7. Jump up and down eight times, then hop on one foot.

8. Name three friends at your school, then walk to the door.

9. Say your age, and then say your friend's age out loud.

10. March to the end of the room, then raise your arm.

12-unit/word lengths

1. Say your full name and draw a tree next to a house.

2. With a pen, write your name, age, and a friend's full name.

3. Draw a blue chair and a big red ball on a rug.

4. Tell the name of a good food that you like to eat.

5. Skip to the door, see who is there, and clap your hands.

6. Read the first line from a book, then turn the page twice.

7. Place your hands on top of your head and count to ten.

8. Name three things kids like to do when they are not home.

9. Stamp your foot four times and move your head up and down.

10. Name two boys' names that start with T and end with M.

Section 1C:
Following Directions—Delayed Response

Four-unit\word lengths

1. Fold paper after dinner.
2. Drink water before dinner.
3. After dinner, walk outside.
4. At four o'clock, sing.
5. Play games after lunch.

Five-unit\word lengths

1. Before bedtime, brush your teeth.
2. Stamp your feet at noon.
3. Draw a picture before dinner.
4. Say your name during dinner.
5. Put on a coat later.

Six-unit\word lengths

1. Write a long sentence after lunch.
2. Turn on a light after dinner.
3. At 2 o'clock, wash your hands.
4. Eat a snack before 3 o'clock.
5. Turn on the TV at seven.

Seven-unit\word lengths

1. When it's dark, look out a window.
2. Name two of your friends at noon.
3. Glance through a book at 3 o'clock.
4. Look for a red car after 2.
5. Draw a box and balloon at noon.

Eight-unit\word lengths

1. Two hours after lunch, sit on the sofa.
2. An hour before dinner, draw a blue bird.
3. Put a toy under your bed at noon.
4. Draw a big black cat after 5 o'clock.
5. At a quarter past two, draw a dog.

Nine-unit\word lengths

1. Put your shoes in a closet at 4 o'clock.

2. After lunch, draw a picture of a pretty house.

3. Say "hi" to a nice person after dinner tonight.

4. Help your best friend with chores before dinner tonight.

5. Straighten one of your dresser drawers after watching TV.

10-unit\word lengths

1. After 12 o'clock, listen to a song, then eat lunch.

2. After you eat dinner, name the color you like best.

3. Before 4 o'clock, put on a hat while you smile.

4. Talk with a friend and solve a problem before bedtime.

5. Open your mouth and blink your eyes after 5 o'clock.

11-unit\word lengths

1. After 2 o'clock, take off your shoes, then clap your hands.

2. After lunch, draw pictures of a small bird and a cat.

3. Make your bed, comb your hair, and smile before breakfast tomorrow.

4. At four o'clock, tell the name of a food you like.

5. Look out the window, then touch the floor before seven o'clock.

12-unit/word lengths

1. Move two pencils from the table to the chair after seven o'clock.

2. After lunch, draw a box, then color it with a green crayon.

3. Put your hands on your head, then stamp your feet at noon.

4. On white lined paper, write your name and age after eight o'clock.

5. Turn on a light and say your name out loud at noon.

Four-unit\word lengths

1. Describe two holiday traditions.

2. Name reasons to exercise.

3. Write your middle name.

4. Erase your last name.

5. Circle your first name.

Five-unit\word lengths

1. Recite the alphabet two times.

2. Turn your left wrist quickly.

3. Spell a three-syllable word.

4. Ask someone for the date.

5. Look for a black stapler.

Six-unit\word lengths

1. Remove two pencils from the desk.

2. Request the time, day, and date.

3. Select three crayons from the box.

4. Open a book to page 30.

5. Fold a paper into three parts.

Seven-unit\word lengths

1. Snap your fingers before you stand up.

2. Rub your hands after you cough twice.

3. Yawn three times and then smile once.

4. Open and shut the drawer three times.

5. Fold a white envelope into four quarters.

Eight-unit\word lengths

1. Look up at four corners of the room.

2. Smile, cough, and scratch your head two times.

3. Say your phone number backward and then forward.

4. Name the seven days of the week twice.

5. Spell your first name, then your last name.

Nine-unit\word lengths

1. Name and write the five vowels of the alphabet.

2. Name three TV shows on Tuesday or Thursday evenings.

3. Cover half your left hand with your right hand.

4. Name two radio stations that play soft rock music.

5. Draw a big orange box on a pink house.

10-unit\word lengths

1. Write your phone number on a small piece of paper.

2. Wiggle the fingers on your left hand while you smile.

3. Clap your hands five times before you stamp your feet.

4. Spell *apartment* and tell how many syllables are in it.

5. Draw the face of a cartoon character on lined paper.

11-unit\word lengths

1. Cover the right-hand corner of this page with your left hand.

2. Name the seasons of the year with the exception of winter.

3. Count the number of windows in the room nearest to you.

4. Tell why it is important to be careful when crossing streets.

5. Name two countries in Europe in which Spanish is not spoken.

12-unit\word lengths

1. Name three odd numbers and four even numbers under the number 20.

2. Tell in which western state the city of San Francisco is located.

3. Draw a small triangle inside a medium square inside a large circle.

4. Fold a small piece of paper into four equal parts, then cough.

5. Clap your hands before you touch your nose and scratch your ear.

Four-unit\word lengths

1. Watch the news tonight.
2. Drink milk at dinner.
3. Recall four commercials later.
4. Wash your face soon.
5. Call a friend tonight.

Five-unit\word lengths

1. Eat a salad with dinner.
2. Help Mom clear the table.
3. Set your alarm by 9:00.
4. Read two newspaper articles soon.
5. Straighten one desk drawer later.

Six-unit\word lengths

1. Straighten the dresser drawer by 8.
2. Brush your teeth at 9 o'clock.
3. Read a short story after dinner.
4. List chores for the week tonight.
5. Write a thank-you note at 6.

Seven-unit\word lengths

1. Recopy your homework assignments at 5 o'clock.
2. Finish all your homework by 8 o'clock.
3. Offer to help Mom with chores tonight.
4. Call a friend at 7 o'clock tonight.
5. Draw a picture of a tree later.

Eight-unit\word lengths

1. Turn on the radio and TV at 5.
2. Take off your shoes before you eat dinner.
3. Put on a hat after you eat lunch.
4. Sing the song you like best at noon.
5. Draw a red dot in a square tonight.

Nine-unit\word lengths

1. Finish your homework before you watch TV this evening.
2. Read a newspaper article about the president this morning.
3. Organize what clothes you'll wear tomorrow by 8 o'clock.
4. Call a friend on the telephone at 7 o'clock.
5. Thank someone for a recent favor at 9 o'clock.

10-unit\word lengths

1. Carry the newspapers out to the garbage at 7 o'clock.
2. Make a peanut butter and jelly sandwich at 4 o'clock.
3. Examine a map of the United States sometime this evening.
4. Straighten your sock drawer and dust your dresser this afternoon.
5. Do four sit-ups and two leg raises at 5 o'clock.

11-unit\word lengths

1. Make a list of chores for next week by dinner time.
2. Wash the bathroom sink and straighten one desk drawer by evening.
3. At 7 p.m., watch the news and remember two important stories.
4. Help a family member with a kitchen chore before bedtime tonight.
5. Select which clothes you plan to wear tomorrow at 9 o'clock.

12-unit\word lengths

1. Remember to brush your teeth and wash your face at 8 o'clock.
2. Read an article from today's newspaper and write a brief summary tonight.
3. Write a short note to a friend describing an upcoming event tonight.
4. Before dinner, read the TV schedule and choose two shows to watch.
5. After 2 p.m., ask Mother if she needs any help before dinner.

Task Accuracy Form

Use this form to document progress for a variety of procedures.

Task Accuracy

Student:				Section:
Sentence Group:				Date:

	Trial #1	Trial #2	Trial #3	Trial #4	Trial #5
1.					
2.					
3.					
4.					
5.					
6.					
7.					
8.					
9.					
10.					

Central Auditory Processing Disorder / Dorothy A. Kelly, D.A. / ISBN 0761631623

Section 2:
Auditory Discrimination

The contrasts described in "On Improving Auditory Discrimination Skills" (see page 142) are designed to improve the ability to identify various phoneme pairs as *same* or *different*. When presenting these contrasts, vary rates, volume, and other factors according to individual needs. This type of exercise is related to the more comprehensive activities which follow (see pages 195-214).

If the child experiences considerable difficulty with discriminating any or all single-phoneme contrasts, you may choose to eliminate that aspect of the program and proceed with other materials.

The auditory discrimination activities that follow are varied in nature and incorporate a broad language-based focus. Generally they begin with easier tasks and progress in degree of challenge. Not all children with CAPD will be able to complete the tasks effectively.

The activities often cross the technical boundaries of "auditory discrimination" into other related areas such as "auditory perception" as described by Gillet (1993, 51-52). When discrimination skills complement other language-based skills, they become more functional.

As with all the materials presented in this chapter, these activities are meant to be representative rather than comprehensive. When the child can participate in creating materials, it adds to the breadth of language.

Skill Area: Auditory Discrimination

Title: Long Vowels

Part 1. Present each long vowel sound in isolation, and then in association with its written symbol and alphabet letter name. Randomly produce various vowel phonemes, and ask the child to identify each one heard by pointing to its written symbol. Repeat this procedure 15 times. Then reverse the process, with the child producing 10 stimulus phonemes while you respond.

Explain the use of /y/ as a vowel sound in both this lesson and the lesson on short vowels (page 213).

a	e	i	o	u

Part 2. Read the following words in random order, and ask the child to identify which long vowel sound is heard in the initial position. Then ask the child to compose a similar list of 10 sets of words.

ate	odor	opal	_____
eat	easy	utility	_____
ice cream	enough	universe	_____
usual	idle	ideas	_____
opener	use	ape	_____
universe	eel	April	_____
over	oatmeal	utilize	_____
island	acorn	evil	_____
aid	ivy	icicle	_____
icon	ache	oak	_____

Part 3. Ask the child to underline the following word sequences (or repeat them) in the order that they are heard. Read the words aloud in random order. Make contrasts between long and short vowel sounds.

This lesson and the lesson entitled Short Vowels (page 213) may be used in combination, with elements from both lessons blended. Ask the child to compose and write original 10-word sequences.

open universe	_____	eel odor	_____
use ideas	_____	eat acorns	_____
over ice	_____	oval island	_____
idle apes	_____	ate ice cream	_____
enough aid	_____	usual ivy	_____

Skill Area: Auditory Discrimination

Title: Compound Words

Part 1. Read words in random order from each of the following groups of two-syllable, compound (and equally emphasized) words. Ask the child to identify the word heard by pointing to it in written form or repeating it, depending on individual needs. Explain that such words are spoken with equal emphasis (similar lengths, pitches, and volumes). Work with the child to create an original list of words (Column D). Use the list for reading, writing, spelling, speaking, and memory activities.

A	B	C	D
sidewalk	something	doorbell	_____
baseball	township	tonight	_____
football	Sunday	bluebird	_____
cowboy	checkbook	sunshine	_____
railroad	rainfall	sunlight	_____
cowgirl	airport	cloudburst	_____
moonlight	cannot	snowshoes	_____
padlock	nightfall	skateboard	_____
makeup	driveway	birthday	_____
workshop	mailroom	backbone	_____

Part 2. Read words from the following lists of multisyllable, compound words. Ask the child to identify each word as it is heard. Point out both the similarities (two words together) as well as the differences between the words (two versus more than two syllables) on this list and the list in Part 1. Work with the child to create an original list of words (Column G).

E	F	G
pullover	dinnerware	_____
afternoon	summertime	_____
newspaper	typewriter	_____
grandfather	whatsoever	_____
grandmother	weatherproofing	_____
grandparent	dishwasher	_____
crybaby	turnover	_____
strawberry	boysenberries	_____
anything	whenever	_____
grasshopper	whatever	_____

Skill Area: Auditory Discrimination

Title: Word Bases

Part 1. Read the following words in random order. Ask the child to point to, repeat, or number the words in the order that they are heard. Use these groups of words to reinforce speaking, reading, spelling, memory, vowel identification, and sentence construction skills. Emphasize the concept of rhyming, and use examples in poems. Have the child create three groups of word bases and read them aloud while you respond.

_____at	_____ike	_____us(s)	_____
bat	bike	bus	
fat	hike	fuss	
hat	like	muss	
mat	Mike	Russ	
sat	pike	Gus	

_____in	_____ed	_____eed	_____
kin	fed	need	
fin	Ned	weed	
pin	led	feed	
tin	wed	breed	
win	red	heed	

_____ow	_____ot	_____use	_____
low	cot	refuse	
grow	not	fuse	
flow	hot	abuse	
row	dot	amuse	
slow	rot	accuse	

Part 2. Read the following word sequences, and ask the child to underline or repeat each as it is heard. Ask the child to construct five original sequences. Emphasize the differences between a sequence and a sentence.

1. Mike's tin pin
2. led the red bike
3. not a hot pot
4. a low row
5. like Russ's bus

6. _____
7. _____
8. _____
9. _____
10. _____

Skill Area: Auditory Discrimination

Title: Verb Endings

Part 1. Read words in random order from the following groups. Ask the child to point to or repeat each word as it is heard. Emphasize the concepts of word bases and tense markers.

Use these groups for syllabication and vowel identification exercises, auditory memory, reading, spelling, sentence constructions, and speech activities.

dress	walk	carry	mow
dressed	walked	carried	mowed
dresses	walks	carries	mows
dressing	walking	carrying	mowing
play	growl	climb	spill
played	growled	climbed	spilled
plays	growls	climbs	spills
playing	growling	climbing	spilling
fix	frighten	grin	switch
fixed	frightened	grinned	switched
fixes	frightens	grins	switches
fixing	frightening	grinning	switching
enjoy	trick	remember	ask
enjoyed	tricked	remembered	asked
enjoys	tricks	remembers	asks
enjoying	tricking	remembering	asking
thank	paint	hurry	iron
thanked	painted	hurried	ironed
thanks	paints	hurries	irons
thanking	painting	hurrying	ironing

(continued)

Part 2. Read the following sentence pairs. Ask the child to underline (or repeat) the sentence heard. Then ask the child to construct two similar sentence pairs and read them aloud, while you respond.

1. The dog growled.

   The dog is growling.

2. She remembers the play.

   She will remember the play.

3. She mows the grass.

   She mowed the grass.

4. He asks the teacher questions.

   He asked the teacher questions.

5. They are painting all the walls today.

   They will paint all the walls today.

6. _____

   _____

7. _____

   _____

Skill Area: Auditory Discrimination

Title: /r/ and /w/

Part 1. Read the following words aloud. Ask the child to either write or say "R" or "W" depending on whether an /r/ or /w/ was heard anywhere in the word. Ask the child to indicate both letters if both sounds were heard. Point out that /r/ tends to be longer in duration than /w/.

For a variation, ask the child to indicate particular positions of the sound (for example, "R in the initial position").

Ask the child to think of 10 examples for you to identify.

window	_____
carpet	_____
rare	_____
wind	_____
battery	_____
chairperson	_____
wouldn't	_____
waterway	_____
wristwatch	_____
weatherperson	_____

Part 2. Read the following word pairs aloud. Ask the child to indicate "same" or "different" for each pair. Then ask the child to compose five word pairs for you to identify.

rater-waiter	ripe-ripe	_____
went-rent	ray-way	_____
west-rest	wail-rail	_____
rare-rare	ride-ride	_____
run-one	west-west	_____

Part 3. Ask the child to point to or number the word sequences in the order heard.

a rare wit	_____
the wide rail	_____
rake and weeds	_____
wailing and weeping	_____
running and riding	_____

Skill Area: Auditory Discrimination

Title: Word Groups

Part 1. Read the following word groups aloud in random order. Ask the child to identify each word by pointing to it and/or repeating it. Not all groups are centered around root bases. For example, some are focused around common vowel sounds or consonant blends. Point out the common base of each group, and provide other helpful information such as irregular spellings, vowel sounds, etc. Use this list for spelling, auditory memory sequence, sentence construction, and other activities.

ai	air	ay	br	ck	ea
train	hair	play	break	sick	eat
rain	stair	gray	brand	pack	read
paint	pair	pray	breeze	stick	cream
chain	lair	sway	breath	stack	least
remain	repair	tray	branch	duck	feast
daily	chair	clay	bring	lock	yeast
afraid	air	jay	bridge	crack	cheat
brain	flair	away	brick	stock	seal
nail	affair	relay	brave	black	beat
stain	fair	stray	bristle	knock	heat

ew	gr	ir	kn	nk	oi
new	grow	girl	know	think	boil
blew	grand	first	knight	thank	point
grew	greet	firm	knew	drank	toil
flew	grate	flirt	knock	prank	spoil
stew	grave	circus	known	honk	avoid
few	ground	circumference	knee	bank	void
jewel	grain	thirst	knit	plank	coil
crew	group	squirm	knot	pink	noise
drew	grasp	skirt	knowledge	trunk	moist
screw	grown	shirt	knife	bunk	voice

(continued)

Word Groups (continued)

or	oo	qu	sp	u	x
corn	look	quit	special	cup	box
born	cook	quaint	spout	up	next
forlorn	book	quest	spell	puddle	mixture
fork	crook	quart	speak	muddle	texture
pork	shook	quite	spin	brush	taxes
north	hook	quiver	spoil	slush	extra
fort	brook	quandary	spoke	shut	express
porter	hood	quicksand	spun	but	six
cork	soot	queen	spook	mutt	fix
horn	good	quake	space	bus	relax

Skill Area: Auditory Discrimination

Title: /f/ and /v/

Part 1. The child with CAPD should use all communication cues, including visual cues. From a speech-reading perspective, /f/ and /v/ are two phonemes that look similar. Because the visual differences between these phonemes is minimal, auditory discrimination training is appropriate. Training will be helpful when distinguishing other confusing contrasts (cognates) as well. Emphasize the difference between the two phonemes in terms of voicing (voiceless/voiced).

Read the following words aloud, and ask the child to indicate whether /f/ or /v/ was heard in the initial position. Ask the child to compose a list of six words to read aloud while you respond.

finger	fortune	fastening	_____
fire	vest	villa	_____
vase	van	vanilla	_____
value	vacuum	foot	_____
vacation	Vincent	foolish	_____
finally	factor	Vanessa	_____

Part 2. Ask the child to listen for only the /v/ sound and indicate its position (initial, medial, or final) in the following words.

relative	remove
vegetables	explosive
villagers	marvelous
velvet	beaver
believe	inventions

Part 3. Ask the child to listen for only the /f/ sound and indicate its position (initial, medial, or final). Afterward, identify odd spellings for the /f/ sound (*gh, ph*).

roughhouse	cough
stuffing	Philadelphia
coffee	fluff
fantastic	baffle
finally	confusing

(continued)

/f/ and /v/ (continued)

Part 4. Ask the child to indicate whether /f/, /v/, or neither sound was heard in any position in the following words. Then ask the child to compose a list of five words and read them aloud while you respond.

laughing   _____

Beverly   _____

revealing   _____

successful   _____

responsible   _____

Part 5. Ask the child to number the following word pairs in the order heard. Read the word pairs aloud in random order.

thief's valentine   _____

thieves' valentines   _____

belief in values   _____

believes in values   _____

firefighters cough   _____

firefighters coughing   _____

stuffed vegetables   _____

stuffing vegetables   _____

Skill Area: Auditory Discrimination

Title: ch and sh

Part 1. Identify both ch and sh in isolation and then associate each blend with its written form. Ask the child to identify each one several times as it is produced. Then ask the child to listen to the following groups of words and identify whether a ch or sh has been produced. Use the same list to randomly produce words, and ask the child to number the words in the order heard. Encourage the child to repeat the words as they are heard. Ask the child to compose additional lists.

For a variation, read the words in random order and have the child identify the blend as well as the position (initial, medial, or final) for each word.

Use these lists for spelling and sentence construction exercises.

Initial Position

_____ chicken	_____ shade
_____ shoe	_____ ship
_____ child	_____ children
_____ choose	_____ shoot
_____ should	_____ cheese

Medial Position

_____ matches	_____ witches
_____ sunshine	_____ washing
_____ cushion	_____ switches
_____ speeches	_____ scratching
_____ milk shake	_____ riches

Final Position

_____ catch	_____ smash
_____ wash	_____ peach
_____ screech	_____ beach
_____ latch	_____ fresh
_____ crush	_____ wish

(continued)

ch and sh (continued)

Part 2. Read the following word groups in random order, and ask the child to identify the word sequences in the order heard. Then ask the child to compose five word sequences.

screeching children   _____

pushing chairs   _____

choose milk shakes   _____

seashore sunshine   _____

changing shirts   _____

Skill Area: Auditory Discrimination

Title: /s/ and /z/

Part 1. Present and contrast the sounds of /s/ and /z/ in isolation. Point out that the sounds differ only in voicing, and that other cues such as duration or length are similar. Identify the names of the letters, their written forms, and their sounds. Ask the child to identify the following word pairs as "same" or "different." Explain that the /s/ or /z/ sounds can be heard in any position in the words. Ask the child to identify how the words are different (for example, /s/ versus /z/ at the end of a word). Ask the child to compose five word pairs to ask you.

bus-buzz	lassie-lazy	_____
sipper-zipper	graze-grass	_____
soon-zoom	has-has	_____
zest-zest	zap-sap	_____
muscle-muzzle	craze-craze	_____

Part 2. Ask the child to indicate whether /s/ or /z/ (or both or neither) is heard in any position in the following words. Remind the child to listen for the sound and not necessarily think of how the word is spelled.

orchestra	zigzag
wasn't	zones
messages	condition
unsolved	understand

Part 3. Read the following aloud. Ask the child to number the word sequences in the order that they are heard. Ask the child to compose five sequences to read aloud while you respond.

lazy muscles	_____
wasn't sooner	_____
unsolved messages	_____
grazing grass	_____
crazy lassie	_____

Part 4. Have the child choose any words from the lists above and use them in silly sentences.

Skill Area: Auditory Discrimination

Title: /m/ and /n/

Part 1. Introduce /m/ and /n/ in isolation. Then correlate each sound with its written form. Contrast and compare both sounds in terms of articulation, nasal resonance, duration, and so on. Present pairs of sounds, and ask the children to say whether they are "same" or "different." Ask the child to listen to the following words and identify where in the word (initial, medial, or final position) the /m/ sound is heard. Ask the child to compose a list of five words and read them aloud while you respond.

mine	armies	middle	_____
jump	dreaming	animals	_____
ram	moonlight	sometimes	_____
swim	aims	comb	_____
movie	cream	cucumber	_____

Part 2. Repeat the exercise in Part 1, using the /n/ sound.

begin	anteaters	plant	_____
hunting	morning	cannot	_____
teenagers	afternoon	nimbus	_____
next	corn	drank	_____
found	learning	cinder	_____

Part 3. Ask the child to listen to the following words and indicate whether /m/ or /n/ (or both or neither) is heard in any position of each word. Ask the child to compose a list of 15 words to read aloud while you respond. Use these lists for spelling, reading, and syllabication exercises.

small	orange	schoolroom
third	mopping	pencil
officer	assignment	newsman
Kentucky	congressperson	principal
telephones	million	fortieth

Part 4. Use at least ten of the words above to write a paragraph about school. Ask the child to read the paragraph aloud while you raise your hand each time one of the words is heard. Then reverse the procedure and ask the child to listen.

Skill Area: Auditory Discrimination

Title: th (voiceless) and wh

Part 1. Present th and wh in isolation, associating sounds with written forms. Contrast both sounds in several "same or different" exercises. Point out that th may also be voiced (as in the word *them*).

Read the following words aloud, and ask the child to indicate which sound was heard in the beginning of each word. Ask the child to compose a list of five words to read aloud while you respond.

Use this list for spelling and sentence construction exercises.

think	whisk	_____
whistle	thimble	_____
thin	thick	_____
thank	which	_____
white	wheelbarrow	_____

Part 2. Read the following words aloud, and ask the child to count the number of syllables in each word and indicate whether th or wh is heard in any position.

nothing	mothballs
fifth	Thanksgiving
whaling	meanwhile
whenever	healthier
something	whiter

Part 3. Read the following words in random order, and ask the child to number the words in the order that they are heard. Ask the child to compose a list of 10 words and read them aloud while you respond.

whistles	thimbles	_____	_____
withering	whistleblower	_____	_____
whalebone	nineteenth	_____	_____
thicknesses	whatsoever	_____	_____
withholding	whine	_____	_____

Part 4. Ask the child to create a story containing any 10 of the words listed above. Ask the child to read the story aloud while you identify words that contain either sound as they are heard. Then create another story, and ask the child to identify the words that contain either sound.

Skill Area: Auditory Discrimination

Title: /k/ and x

Part 1. Identify /k/ and x in isolation, and associate each with its sound and written forms. Contrast both sounds, and ask the child to identify several pairs as "same" or "different." Point out that the sound of /k/ is sometimes spelled with a c (as in the word *cat*).

Read the following words aloud, and ask the child to identify the /k/ (or /c/) sound as being in the initial, medial, or final position in each word. Ask the child to compose a list of 10 words to read aloud while you respond.

Use these words in syllabication, spelling, and sentence construction exercises.

1. kettle	6. package	_____	_____
2. bookcase	7. crackle	_____	_____
3. keyboard	8. bleak	_____	_____
4. wreck	9. macaroni	_____	_____
5. trick-or-treat	10. kangaroo	_____	_____

Part 2. Repeat Part 1, using the x sound. Point out that the sound of x is similar to a /ks/ sound.

1. extra	6. axis	_____	_____
2. relax	7. flexible	_____	_____
3. oxen	8. waxen	_____	_____
4. fox	9. taxing	_____	_____
5. axe	10. maximum	_____	_____

Part 3. Randomly select words from both groups above, and ask the child to identify which sound was heard and in what position.

Part 4. Randomly select words, and ask the child to identify the word sequences heard. Ask the child to compose one pair of word sequences to read aloud while you respond.

1. fixing wrecks
   picking wrecks

2. flexible cake pan
   king-size cake pan

3. meeker boxer
   kinder boxer

4. likes taxis
   likes cases

5. tax cities
   fax cities

6. _____
   _____

Skill Area: Auditory Discrimination

Title: /p/ and /t/

Part 1. Present /p/ and /t/ in isolation, and then associate each with sound and written forms. Contrast the two phonemes as "same" or "different."

Read the following word pairs aloud, and ask the child to identify them as "same" or "different." All words used have either a /p/ or /t/ in the initial position and possibly elsewhere as well.

Ask the child to compose five word pairs and read them aloud for you to identify as "same" or "different."

page-page	teacher-preacher	_____
Tuesday-Tuesday	preacher-preacher	_____
pen-ten	pile-tile	_____
tot-top	tea-pea	_____
puppy-putty	test-pest	_____

Part 2. Read the following words aloud, and ask the child to identify which sound (or sounds) are heard in any position and tell the number of syllables. Ask the child to compose another list of five words for you to identify.

secretive	sedimentary	_____
telegraphic	computerized	_____
territories	Mississippi	_____
peaceful	respectable	_____
protective	repetitious	_____

Part 3. Ask the child to create a story containing any 10 of the above words. Ask the child to read the story aloud while you raise your hand whenever one of the words is heard. Then reverse roles: create another story, read it aloud, and ask the child to raise a hand whenever one of the words is heard.

Part 4. Dictate the following word pairs while the child spells them and names the number of syllables heard.

present

prideful

trillion

tactic

inflatable

Skill Area: Auditory Discrimination

Title: Short Vowels

Part 1. Identify each of the short vowel sounds in isolation by alphabet name, written symbol, and sound. Ask the child to similarly identify each vowel and write each one on a sheet of paper. Randomly produce the sounds of each vowel, and ask the child to identify them. Briefly contrast the short vowels with long vowels. Explain the use of /y/ as a vowel sound in both this lesson and the lesson on long vowels (page 195).

a   e   i   o   u

Part 2. Read the following word pairs aloud, and ask the child to identify each pair as "same" or "different."

slap-slop	_____	hit-hot	_____
pass-pass	_____	cup-cup	_____
add-odd	_____	tip-top	_____
map-mop	_____	bend-bend	_____
chop-chop	_____	rest-rust	_____

Part 3. Read the following words aloud, and ask the child to listen for the short /i/ sound and identify whether it is in the initial, medial, or final position. (Some words do not contain the sound.) Ask the child to compose a list of five words to read aloud while you respond.

him	pumpkin	_____
continue	kitten	_____
invite	settle	_____
cupcake	listen	_____
ribbon	mission	_____

Part 4. Repeat Part 3, using the short /o/ sound.

otter	disk	_____
clockwise	olives	_____
oval	opportunity	_____
floppy	message	_____
computer	octagon	_____

For a variation, repeat the activities in Part 3 and Part 4, using the remaining short vowel sounds.

(continued)

Short Vowels (continued)

Part 5. Read the following word sequences, and ask the child to number them in the order they are heard. Ask the child to compose five word sequences and read them aloud while you respond.

rotten eggs   _____

hopping bunny   _____

which insects   _____

timid animals   _____

silly friends   _____

Section 3:
Auditory Cohesion

Skill Area: Auditory Cohesion

Title: Similarities and Differences

Part 1. Read each of the following paired words aloud, and ask the child to identify attributes or characteristics that are same and different. Not all of the pairs contain the names of objects. Ask the child to repeat the paired words aloud once before responding. More than one response may be correct. After each response, ask the child to explain why the response was made. Identify why the response was correct or incorrect (for example, "It seems that you thought _____ because _____"). Dictate any two of the pairs and ask the child to write down the dictation. Encourage the child to use note-taking skills (see page 161) to complete this task.

1. cookies/cakes

2. air conditioner/electric heater

3. dog/horse

4. snow/rain

5. smoke/clouds

6. flour/sand

7. car/train

8. ten/thirty

9. pretty/handsome

10. neat/messy

11. _____

12. _____

Part 2—Turnaround. Ask the child to compose five paired combinations and read them aloud while you respond, explaining why each attribute or characteristic was paired (for example, "I think _____ because _____"). The child confirms the logic or lack of logic for each response. Then the child writes down any two of these pairs. Encourage the child to use proofreading skills (see page 163) to check the writing. The child then reads the paired combinations aloud.

1. _____

2. _____

3. _____

4. _____

5. _____

Skill Area: Auditory Cohesion

Title: Conversations

Part 1. Ask the child to identify suitable endings to the conversations provided below. Ask the child to repeat the conversation aloud once before responding. After each response, ask the child to explain the response. More than one response may be correct. Identify why the response was correct or incorrect (for example, "Did you say _____ because you thought that _____?").

Ask the child to identify who the conversational partners might be (for example, a mother and her child) as well as how each partner might be feeling. Dictate any two of the conversations and ask the child to write down the dictation. Encourage the child to use note-taking skills (see page 161) to complete this task.

This lesson has apparent pragmatic implications.

1. A: Hi! How are you?

   B: Fine. How are you doing?

   A: Terrific! Where are you going?

   B: . . .

2. A: I just found out that I failed my social studies test.

   B: Oh, that's too bad. Did you forget to study?

   A: No, I studied all right. It was something else.

   B: . . .

3. A: This is my new puppy.

   B: Oh, she's so cute. Where did you get her?

   A: We got her in the pet store at the mall.

   B: . . .

4. A: Where do you want to go today?

   B: I don't know. Where do you want to go?

   A: How about seeing a movie?

   B: . . .

5. A: I'm too tired to clean the house today.

   B: Can I help?

   A: Thanks! Will you wash the floor?

   B: . . .

(continued)

6. A: I need five more dollars for the game I want to buy.

   B: Well, why don't you do some extra work and earn the money?

   A: No. I hate to do chores.

   B: . . .

7. A: Every time I want to watch a TV show, you won't let me.

   B: Don't you think that's a little bit of an exaggeration?

   A: What I mean is, all my friends watch more TV than I do.

   B: . . .

8. A: Where is my homework?

   B: I haven't seen it. Where were you doing your homework last night?

   A: What does that have to do with anything?

   B: . . .

9. A: Are you going to Sean's party?

   B: I didn't even know that he was having a party.

   A: Yes, he is. It's next Saturday.

   B: . . .

10. A: May I help you?

    B: Yes. I'm looking for a present for my father.

    A: How much do you want to spend?

    B: . . .

For a variation, continue the conversations further. Ask the child to create two inappropriate responses and explain why they are inappropriate.

11. _____

12. _____

Part 2—Turnaround. Ask the child to produce five conversations and read them aloud while you respond and explain each conversation ending (for example, "I think _____ because _____"). Ask the child to confirm the logic or lack of logic for each ending. Then ask the child to write down any two of these conversations. Encourage the child to use proofreading skills (see page 163) to check the writing. Then ask the child to read the conversations aloud.

1. _____   4. _____

2. _____   5. _____

3. _____

Skill Area: Auditory Cohesion

Title: Verbal Math Problems

Part 1. Read each of the following math problems aloud, and ask the child to identify logical methods (for example, "Divide 25 by 4") to solve each one. Encourage the child to repeat the problem aloud once before responding. More than one method may be correct. After each response, ask the child to explain the response. Identify why the response was correct or incorrect (for example, "It seems that you said _____ because _____"). Dictate any two of the problems and ask the child to write down the dictation. Encourage the child to use note-taking skills (see page 161) to complete this task.

1. You made 54 cookies for your class. There are 22 students in class. How may cookies did each student get?

2. You are allowed to watch 10 hours of television each week. There are two movies that you want to see on Sunday. Each one is 2 hours long. How many hours of time will you have left for the rest of the week?

3. You want to buy your mother a birthday gift for $12.00. You receive $2.00 a week in allowance. You have $4.00 saved already. How many more weeks must you save?

4. Your dog costs $1.25 a day to feed. How much does it cost to feed him for a full year?

5. Your sister gave you $5.00, your father gave you $11.00, and your uncle gave you $20.00. You gave your brother $6.00, and you had $15.00 of your own. How much money do you have?

6. You want to carpet your room, which is 12 feet by 18 feet in size. How many square yards of carpet must you buy?

7. How many odd numbers are between 8 and 50?

8. You have a food budget of $200.00 for the month. How much money could you spend on food each week? How much money could you spend for a half-year?

9. Your car can travel 25 miles on one gallon of gas. You want to go on a 375-mile trip. How many gallons of gas will you need?

10. Your house is 30 feet high. Your garage is 21 feet high. Your doghouse is 4 feet high. How much taller is your garage than your doghouse?

11. _____

   _____

12. _____

   _____

(continued)

Verbal Math Problems (continued)

Part 2—Turnaround. Ask the child to create five verbal math problems and read them aloud while you respond and explain the method used to solve each problem (for example, "I think _____ because _____"). Ask the child to confirm the logic or lack of logic for each response. Then ask the child to write down any two of the problems. Encourage the child to use proofreading skills (see page 163) to check the writing. Then ask the child to read the problems aloud.

For a variation of either Part 1 or Part 2, include a fact in each problem that is not necessary to solve it. For example, in #10, the height of the house was not needed. Ask the child to identify the unnecessary information.

1. _____

   _____

2. _____

   _____

3. _____

   _____

4. _____

   _____

5. _____

   _____

Skill Area: Auditory Cohesion

Title: Story Titles

Part 1. Ask the child to create a suitable title for each of the mini-stories below. Ask the child to repeat the story aloud once before responding. After each response, ask the child to explain the response. More than one response may be correct. Identify why the response was correct or incorrect (for example, "Did you say _____ because you thought that _____?").

Dictate any two of the stories and ask the child to write down the dictation. Encourage the child to use note-taking skills (see page 161) to complete this task.

1. John moved to a new neighborhood. He didn't know anyone. On the first day of school, he felt very shy. The day went so slowly.

2. Six friends won the lottery last month. They decided to split the money evenly and go on a fantastic vacation. Each person named a place to go.

3. Chris was doing poorly in math this year. He really hadn't spent enough time on homework or studying. Just before his final exam, he had a change of heart. He studied four hours for the test and did two extra-credit projects.

4. Jenny was thirteen years old. She wanted to do something important during her summer vacation. She decided to act as a "big sister" to a little girl in her neighborhood who was having some problems at school.

5. It was two days before Josh's mother's birthday, and he wanted to surprise her. He called her sister, who lived in a distant state, and asked her for some ideas. His aunt came up with a terrific suggestion.

6. Sam became very tired of reading all the negative stories in his local newspaper. He decided to keep a journal of all the positive events that occurred during one month. At the end of the month, he sent his journal to the editor of the newspaper.

7. Lauren became very discouraged about house-training her new puppy. Her parents were considering returning it to the puppy store if matters didn't improve within the next week. Lauren came up with a creative method of getting the point across to the puppy.

8. The seventh-grade girls' basketball team was challenged to a game by the eighth-grade team at a neighboring school. Although they had a record of 7 wins and 2 losses so far that season, they weren't sure whether they should accept the challenge.

9. The new principal at school seemed to be strict. She implemented a new dress code for all students on her very first day. The students wanted to cooperate, but felt that the code was a little harsh.

10. Mike became very tired of being the "class clown." He realized that it took a great deal of energy to keep the class entertained. He also realized that the attention he was getting from his teachers was not the kind that he really wanted. He decided to make a change.

(continued)

Story Titles (continued)

For a variation, ask the child to create an appropriate ending for any of the stories above.

11. _____

_____

12. _____

_____

Part 2—Turnaround. Ask the child to create five stories and read or tell them aloud while you respond and explain why you chose each title and ending (for example, "I think _____ because _____"). Ask the child to confirm the logic or lack of logic for each title and ending. Then ask the child to write down any two of the stories. Encourage the child to use proofreading skills (see page 163) to check the writing. Then ask the child to read the stories aloud.

1. _____

_____

2. _____

_____

3. _____

_____

4. _____

_____

5. _____

_____

Skill Area: Auditory Cohesion

Title: Categories

Part 1. Ask the child to name the category for each of the following groups of objects. Ask the child to repeat the names of the category members aloud once before responding. After each response, ask the child to explain the choice. More than one response may be correct. Identify why the response was correct or incorrect (for example, "Did you say _____ because you thought that _____?").

Dictate any two of the groupings and ask the child to write down the dictation. Encourage the child to use note-taking skills (see page 161) to complete this task. Then ask the child to name one additional category member.

This exercise is comparable to Sequences (see page 232), which may be used similarly.

1. Buick, Chevrolet, Toyota, Pontiac, _____

2. San Francisco, Providence, Dallas, Atlanta, _____

3. football, baseball, soccer, tennis, _____

4. lettuce, celery, carrots, tomatoes, _____

5. France, Germany, Spain, Portugal, _____

6. desk, table, sofa, lamp, _____

7. pencils, pens, assignment pad, notebooks, _____

8. teacher, principal, hall monitor, cafeteria worker, _____

9. Thanksgiving, Flag Day, Fourth of July, Memorial Day, _____

10. Lincoln, Washington, Roosevelt, Carter, _____

11. _____

12. _____

Part 2—Turnaround. Ask the child to produce five category groupings and read them aloud while you respond and explain each response (for example, "I said _____ because _____"). Ask the child to confirm the logic or lack of logic for each response. Then ask the child to write down any two of these groupings. Encourage the child to use proofreading skills (see page 163) to check the writing. Then ask the child to read the groupings aloud.

1. _____

2. _____

3. _____

4. _____

5. _____

Skill Area: Auditory Cohesion

Title: Riddles

Part 1. Read the riddles below, and ask the child to respond with logical answers. Ask the child to repeat the riddle aloud once before responding. More than one response may be correct. After each response, ask the child to explain the response. Identify why the response was correct or incorrect (for example, "It seems that you guessed _____ because _____"). Dictate any two of the riddles and ask the child to write down the dictation. Encourage the child to use note-taking skills (see page 161) to complete this task.

Each riddle below begins with, "This is . . ." or "These are . . ." and ends with the question, "What is it?" or "What are they?"

1. This is something that changes color when you add a sweet, dark liquid or powder to it. It originally came from an animal that lives on a farm. What is it? *(milk)*

2. These are things that you wear in snowy weather on your feet. What are they? *(boots)*

3. This is something that usually contains many volumes and is filled with facts and information. What is it? *(encyclopedia)*

4. This is something that can keep you from getting lost. It is made of paper, and it's hard to refold after it's been opened. What is it? *(map)*

5. This is something that has numbers on it and can tell you how much you weigh. What is it? *(scale)*

6. This is an animal that lives with you. You feed it and take it for walks. What is it? *(dog)*

7. These are objects that are small, round in shape, and can be bought in music stores. What are they? *(CDs)*

8. These are publications that usually are delivered to your house once a month and contain stories and pictures. What are they? *(magazines)*

9. This is a building in which people work who deal with deposits and withdrawals of money. What is it? *(bank)*

10. This is a place where you can borrow books. You need a special card with your name on it in order to do this. What is this place? *(library)*

11. _____

_____

12. _____

_____

(continued)

Riddles (continued)

Part 2—Turnaround. Ask the child to create five riddles and read them aloud while you respond and explain each response (for example, "I guessed _____ because _____"). Ask the child to confirm the logic or lack of logic for each response. Ask the child to write down any two of these riddles. Encourage the child to use proofreading skills (see page 163) to check the writing. Then ask the child to read the riddles aloud.

1. _____

_____

2. _____

_____

3. _____

_____

4. _____

_____

5. _____

_____

Skill Area: Auditory Cohesion

Title: Contingencies

Part 1. Ask the child to respond to the following contingency commands. Ask the child to repeat the contingency aloud once before responding. After each response, ask the child to explain the response. Identify why the response was correct or incorrect (for example, "Did you say _____ because you heard the word _____?"). Dictate any two contingency commands and ask the child to write down the dictation. Encourage the child to use note-taking skills (see page 161) to complete this task.

1. If today is the third day of the month, clap your hands. If it is not, touch your nose twice.

2. If you like ice cream less than spinach, count to ten. Otherwise, count to eleven.

3. If you'd rather ride your bike than play video games, name one cartoon character. Otherwise, name your favorite color.

4. If today is colder than it was yesterday and if you like snow, smile. If either one of these things is not true, cough twice.

5. If salad is bad for you, touch your foot. If it isn't, touch both of your ears.

6. If Wednesday is one of the months, stand up. If not, do nothing.

7. If boys are always smarter than girls or if they are always more athletic, look at the floor. If either of these is not true, name the months of the year.

8. If winter and summer are opposites, name your favorite movie. If not, name the president.

9. If a pound of feathers is heavier than a pound of dirt, open your mouth. Otherwise tap your head.

10. If the United States is a country in North America, name your favorite dessert. If it is not, name two cities in your state.

11. _____

    _____

12. _____

    _____

Part 2—Turnaround. Ask the child to produce five contingency commands to ask you. Respond and explain each response (for example, "I _____ because I heard the word _____"). Ask the child to confirm the logic or lack of logic for each response. Ask the child to write down any two of these contingency commands,. Encourage the child to use proofreading skills (see page 163) to check the writing. Then ask the child to read the commands aloud.

1. _____

    _____

2. _____

    _____

Skill Area: Auditory Cohesion

Title: Analogies

Part 1. Read the following analogies aloud, and ask the child to complete each one. Ask the child to repeat the analogy aloud once before responding. After each response, ask the child to explain the response. Identify why the response was correct or incorrect (for example, "Did you say _____ because you heard the word _____?"; or "Did you say _____ because you thought that _____?").

Dictate any two of the analogies and ask the child to write down the dictation. Encourage the child to use note-taking skills (see page 161) to complete this task.

1. Boy is to man as girl is to _____.

2. Cold is to winter as _____ is to summer.

3. Boots are to feet as _____ are to hands.

4. House is to wood as car is to _____.

5. Helicopters are to planes as cars are to _____.

6. Bread is to sandwiches as folders are to _____.

7. Pound is to weight as inch is to _____.

8. Alligator is to reptile as _____ is to mammal.

9. Author is to book as artist is to _____.

10. Telephone is to speech as letters are to _____.

11. _____

12. _____

Part 2—Turnaround. Ask the child to produce five analogies to ask you. Respond and explain each response (for example, "I said _____ because _____"). Ask the child to confirm the logic or lack of logic for each response. Ask the child to write down any two of the analogies. Encourage the child to use proofreading skills (see page 163) to check the writing.

1. _____

2. _____

3. _____

4. _____

5. _____

Skill Area: Auditory Cohesion

Title: Reasoning

Part 1. Read the following questions and ask the child to answer them. Ask the child to repeat the question aloud once before responding. After each response, ask the child to explain the response. Identify why the response was correct or incorrect (for example, "Did you say _____ because you thought that _____?").

Dictate any two of the questions and ask the child to write down the dictation. Encourage the child to use note-taking skills (see page 161) to complete this task.

1. Why is it unfair for a school system to provide more money for boys' sports than for girls' sports?

2. Why is it important to get an education?

3. Why do so many people want to immigrate to the United States?

4. Why should children get allowances?

5. Why should every town have a library?

6. Why is it important for people to vote?

7. Why should everyone learn to read?

8. Why is it important for the United States to have friendly relationships with other countries?

9. Why is it important to have gym classes?

10. Why do many countries throughout the world have school all year round?

11. _____

12. _____

Part 2—Turnaround. Ask the child to produce five questions to ask you. Respond and explain each response (for example, "I said _____ because _____"). Ask the child to confirm the logic or lack of logic for each response. Ask the child to write down any two of the questions. Encourage the child to use proofreading skills (see page 163) to check the writing.

1. _____

2. _____

Skill Area: Auditory Cohesion

Title: Inferences—Questions about People

Part 1. Ask the child to respond to the following questions. Ask the child to repeat the question aloud once before responding. After each response, ask the child to explain the response. Identify why the response was correct or incorrect (for example, "Did you say _____ because you heard the word _____?").

Dictate any two of the questions and ask the child to write down the dictation. Encourage the child to use note-taking skills (see page 161) to complete this task.

1. Who collects money from drivers before they go over bridges?

2. Who is the person whom you never see and who answers questions about phone numbers?

3. Who tells you how much money you have in bank accounts and takes your deposits?

4. Who cuts hair and gives permanents?

5. Who wants to sell you a new car?

6. Who teaches children to play soccer?

7. Who uses a bat and ball and wears a uniform?

8. Who is elected by voters every four years and is the leader of our country?

9. Who keeps the parks clean?

10. Who writes stories every day in the newspapers?

11. _____

12. _____

Part 2—Turnaround. Ask the child to produce five questions to ask you. Respond and explain each response (for example, "I _____ because I heard the word _____"). Ask the child to confirm the logic or lack of logic for each response. Ask the child to write down any two of the questions. Encourage the child to use proofreading skills (see page 163) to check the writing.

1. _____

2. _____

Skill Area: Auditory Cohesion

Title: True or False

Part 1. Ask the child to respond to each of the following statements by indicating whether it is true or false. Ask the child to repeat the statement aloud once before responding. After each response, ask the child to explain the response. Identify why the response was correct or incorrect (for example, "Did you say it was false possibly because you thought that _____?").

Dictate any two of the statements and ask the child to write down the dictation. Encourage the child to use note-taking skills (see page 161) to complete this task.

1. All children who live in this country are Americans.

2. Most people would like to live in Florida.

3. If a person has been elected as president, it means that everyone voted for him or her.

4. You buy socks, shoes, and gloves in pairs.

5. Just because you are old does not mean that you have to stop working.

6. All cities in this country have more than 2 million residents.

7. It is important that all persons graduating from high school go on to college.

8. Computers were invented more than one hundred years ago by a man named Leonardo da Vinci.

9. Encyclopedias and dictionaries are two sources of information.

10. Radios can be powered by batteries or electricity.

11. _____

12. _____

Part 2—Turnaround. Ask the child to produce five statements to ask you. Respond and explain each response (for example, "I said it was true because _____"). Ask the child to confirm the logic or lack of logic for each response. Ask the child to write down any two of the statements. Encourage the child to use proofreading skills (see page 163) to check the writing.

1. _____

2. _____

Skill Area: Auditory Cohesion

Title: Ridiculous Sentences

Part 1. Ask the child to identify what is ridiculous or absurd in the sentences below. Ask the child to repeat the sentence aloud once before responding. After each response, ask the child to explain the response. Identify why the response was correct or incorrect (for example, "Did you say _____ because you heard the word _____?"). Dictate any two of the sentences and ask the child to write down the dictation. Encourage the child to use note- taking skills (see page 161) to complete this task.

1. We like to spend Saturdays at the grocery store reading books.

2. We have had a football game every month except Tuesday so far this week.

3. On Flag Day our family eats turkey, stuffing, cranberries, and pumpkin pie.

4. Whenever the dog whispers, we know that someone is at the door.

5. My studying paid off for the math test—I failed!

6. Whenever I want to cheer myself up, I listen to a sad song.

7. On Mother's Day, I gave my dad some flowers.

8. We saw such beautiful jewelry at the zoo.

9. My letter was returned to me because I remembered to put a stamp on it.

10. I looked at my wrist and realized that I was late for my appointment.

11. _____

12. _____

Part 2—Turnaround. Ask the child to produce five ridiculous statements to present to you. Respond and explain each response (for example, "I _____ because I heard the word _____"). Ask the child to confirm the logic or lack of logic for each response. Ask the child to write down any two of the questions. Encourage the child to use proofreading skills (see page 163) to check the writing.

1. _____

2. _____

Skill Area: Auditory Cohesion

Title: Problem-Solving Choices

Part 1. Read the following situations, and ask the child to identify logical reactions to them. Ask the child to repeat the stimulus question aloud once before responding. After each response, ask the child to explain the response. Identify why the response was correct or incorrect (for example, "It seems that you feel that _____ is a good choice because _____"). Dictate any two of the questions and ask the child to write down the dictation. Encourage the child to use note-taking skills (see page 161) to complete this task.

Begin each question below with "What would you do if . . ."

1. You forgot to study for an important math test?

2. You saw a classmate take an item out of another classmate's desk without permission?

3. You made two appointments at the same time on the same day?

4. You had an argument with a friend and you feel you both were at fault?

5. You lost a library book?

6. You found a wallet with $100.00 in it on the playground?

7. A classmate at school was continually harassing you?

8. You felt that your bedtime was too early?

9. You felt that you had too many chores to do?

10. You missed the late bus at school and you didn't have money to call your parent?

11. _____

12. _____

Part 2—Turnaround. Ask the child to produce five "What if . . .?" questions to ask you. Respond and explain each response (for example, "I would _____ because _____"). Ask the child to confirm the logic or lack of logic for each response. Ask the child to write down any two of the questions. Encourage the child to use proofreading skills (see page 163) to check the writing. Then ask the child to read the questions aloud.

1. _____

2. _____

Skill Area: Auditory Cohesion

Title: Sequences

Part 1. Ask the child to complete each of the following sequences. Ask the child to repeat the sequence aloud once before responding. After each response, ask the child to explain. More than one response may be correct. Identify why the response was correct or incorrect (for example, "Did you say _____ because you thought that _____?").

Dictate any two of the sequences and ask the child to write down the dictation. Encourage the child to use note-taking skills (see page 161) to complete this task.

1. New York, California, Montana, Florida, _____

2. telephones, fax machines, computers, televisions, _____

3. president, senator, congressperson, district attorney, _____

4. oranges, apples, pears, grapes, _____

5. fir, maple, evergreen, oak, _____

6. glue, staples, paper clips, tape, _____

7. books, magazines, newspapers, dictionaries, _____

8. Jennifer, Megan, Laura, Christen, _____

9. geometry, algebra, biology, chemistry, _____

10. dynamite, dessert, diameter, delivery, _____

11. _____

12. _____

Part 2—Turnaround. Ask the child to produce five sequences to ask you. Respond and explain each response (for example, "I said _____ because _____"). Ask the child to confirm the logic or lack of logic for each response. Ask the child to write down any two of the sequences. Encourage the child to use proofreading skills (see page 163) to check the writing. Then ask the child to read the sequences aloud.

1. _____

2. _____

Suggestions for Increasing Overall Auditory Attention

Auditory attention appears to be related in part to other skills (for example, auditory memory and auditory figure-ground) and factors including maturity and interest. The suggestions offered below reflect these influences. You may wish to increase the challenge in these activities in terms of the time involved, setting (front or back of the room, in noise or quiet), degree of participation, or level of language. Provide an incentive that will motivate the child (for example, "If you complete this task successfully as directed, you don't have to do your math homework tonight").

1. Read plays aloud in which the child has an assigned part.

2. Read stories aloud in which the child must listen for specified cue words in order to participate (for example, "Whenever you hear the word _____, you say, '_____' ").

3. Transcribe information from a tape recorder.

4. Ask the child to make a telephone call to someone for a specific purpose (for example, calling mother to get the list of ingredients for a complicated recipe).

5. Ask the child to listen to a radio broadcast or watch a television show until a particular word is heard (for example, "Shut off the television after you have heard the word *woman*").

6. Ask the class or group to build a frightening story by having each child contribute a part in sequence.

7. Ask the child to "listen" to another child's written story in order to help that child discover any errors in content, logic, sentence structure, and so on. Then have the children reverse roles. (Buddy work or cooperative learning should always be of a reciprocated nature.)

8. Ask the child to count how many times a dog barks during a 5-minute tape (or 1, 2, 3, or 4 minutes).

9. Ask the child to listen to a radio broadcast of a baseball game for 5, 10, or more minutes. Afterward, have the child summarize the plays.

10. Ask the child to "help" you in some task that requires attention, such as waiting for an expected phone call or listening for the sounds of the mail carrier.

11. Ask the child to "help" you locate a favorite song on a tape or CD.

12. Play elaborate games that involve auditory cues, such as "Simon Says."

13. Sing songs in which each child in a group sings a specific line or phrase.

14. Ask the child to "be in charge" of listening for such things as fire alarms, public address system announcements, bells for period-changing, and so on.

15. Ask the child to think of ways to increase the ability to maintain auditory attention.

Listening Behaviors

Use this form to document the development of effective listening behaviors. Specifically note negative behaviors such as "interruptions" and "confirmations" (for example, ". . . Right?"). Encourage the child to reduce such behaviors over time. Acquire documentation during a variety of listening tasks, including conversations and classroom lectures.

- -

Listening Behaviors

Child's Name:		Grade/Placement:		
Speech-Language Pathologist:				

Key
A = Interruptions
B = Extraneous physical movements
C = Confirmations
D = Excessive talking during task

Activity:	A	B	C	D
Date:				
Date:				
Date:				
Date:				
Date:				
Date:				
Date:				
Date:				

Central Auditory Processing Disorder / Dorothy A. Kelly, D.A. / ISBN 0761631623

Games

The following games are designed to be "therapy projects" to be completed by the student (or students) over a period of time. Processing skills will be reinforced when the child must analyze and devise tasks as specified.

Traveling by Rocket Ship

Objective: To improve auditory memory, auditory sequential memory, receptive language, and phonics skills

Target Population: Primary-age children with auditory processing disorders

Number of players: Two to four

Materials:

Gameboard (see page 236)

Scissors

Glue

File folder

Crayons or marking pens

Markers (one for each player)

40 3" x 5" index cards

Scissors

Spinner (four sections)

Preparation:

1. Reproduce the gameboard. Trim the edges. Glue the gameboard to the inside of a file folder. Color the gameboard. Laminate it for durability.

2. Cut the index cards in half to make 80 cards, each 3" x 2½" cards. Prepare 20 cards in each of four levels of tasks that vary in degree of difficulty. Instructions can be humorous in nature. Typical cards might be:

   Level #1 (easiest):*

   > Make the /l/ sound.

   > Make the long ā sound.

   > Make the sound of a cow.

   Level #2 (harder):*

   > Repeat these vowels: a . . . e . . . i.

   > Repeat these words that go together: comb . . . brush . . . hair.

---

*Use only single-syllable words in Level #1 and Level #2.

Level #3 (even harder): Give two- or three-step commands or contingencies, such as:

> Stand up, look at the ceiling, and touch your ear.

> If it's raining, then blink your eyes.

Level #4 (hardest): Give four-step commands and/or unrelated sequences to recall four to six units, such as:

> Open your mouth, touch your chin, look out the window, and smile.

> Repeat these words: pencil, window, grass, sky, car.

Playing the Game:

1. Stack the cards in four piles of 20 cards each, according to level of difficulty.

2. Player #1 uses a spinner to determine which stack of cards to draw from.

3. Player #1 draws one card from the indicated stack and reads the instruction to the player on the right.

4. Player #2 carries out the direction correctly and moves the marker as many spaces on the board as designated by the number of the stack (1, 2, 3, or 4).

   If Player #2 lands on a space with a backward arrow, the player moves the marker back 5 spaces.

5. The first player to get back to Earth (the endpoint of the board) wins the game.

Traveling by Rocket Ship

Pluto

Neptune

Uranus

Saturn

Jupiter

Mars

Earth

Venus

Mercury

Central Auditory Processing Disorder / Dorothy A. Kelly, D.A. / ISBN 0761631623

The Sound-It-Out Game

Objective: To improve phonic reading and/or spelling skills

Target Population: Primary school-age children who display reading and/or spelling difficulties

Number of Players: Two to four

Materials:

50 index cards

Scissors

Marking pen

Magnetic or felt letters

Magnetic or felt board

Spinner (four sections)

Preparation:

1. Cut the index cards in half to make 100 3″ x 2½″ cards.

   Prepare 25 cards in each of four levels of words that vary in degree of difficulty. Words on the cards reflect selections from basic vocabulary lists used in schools. Typical cards might be:

   Level #1 (easiest):* Two- or three-sound (or two- or three-letter) words only; for example:

   > h - o - p

   > u - p

   Level #2 (harder):* Four- or five-sound (or four- or five-letter) words only; for example:

   > d - e - s - k

   > c - a - r - d

   Level #3 (even harder): Two-syllable words only; for example:

   > grand - ma

   > rail - way

   Level #4 (hardest): Three-syllable words only; for example:

   > Oc - to - ber

   > re - mem - ber

2. Place the magnetic board on the table, and place the magnetic letters in a pile.

---

*For Level #1 and Level #2, use words that are spelled the way they sound. Format each card in the following manner in order to enable the reader to pronounce the word, sound by sound, as well as to see it in its conventional form:

f–u–n

(fun)

Playing the Game:
1. Stack the cards in four piles of 25 cards each, according to level of difficulty.

2. Player #1 uses the spinner to determine which stack of cards to draw from.

3. Player #1 draws one card from the indicated stack and reads it aloud to the player on the right.

4. Player #2 selects appropriate letters from the pile of letters and places them on the felt or magnetic board to spell the word on the card. Player #2 then says the word. Player #1 checks the accuracy of the effort. If the word is spelled and produced correctly, Player #2 is awarded one point per letter.

5. The first player to acquire 100 points wins the game.

Simon Says

Simon Says has many applications for children with central auditory processing disorder. It can be used to improve auditory memory and the ability to interpret directions by presenting complicated or multipart commands. It also can be used to improve auditory discrimination/perception by including "error" words in the direction (for example, "Clap your arms three times"). It can be useful to build auditory attention by increasing the overall playing time and/or by increasing the child's participation in the game. It may even be useful in improving auditory figure-ground skills if the game is played with background noise.

Turnaround benefits may be derived by having the child construct the directions, either writing them independently or by having them dictated and then reading them aloud.

Playing the Game:

The following examples may be used to begin the game.

1. Simon says, "Touch both ears."

2. Simon says, "Look out the window."

3. Sit down.

4. Wiggle your fingers.

5. Shake your head.

6. Simon says, "Close your eyes and open your mouth."

7. Simon says, "Tap your left knee four times."

8. Simon says, "Turn your left shoulder toward the door."

9. Simon says, "Jump two times."

10. Point to your right foot.

11. _____

12. _____

PART FIVE

Transition and Carryover

While Part Four focused on specific therapy materials, Part Five is concerned with follow-up in various forms. Once the child has completed the CAPD program, the clinician may suggest different ways to monitor and maintain skill levels. Chapter 9 provides sample letters to parents, physicians, and audiologists, as well as a form for Discharge from Therapy.

9

Transition and Carryover Concerns

From Therapy to Independence

Therapy does not end at the point of discharge for children with central auditory processing disorder. It simply metamorphoses into a more informal, self-regulated format. In many cases, CAPD appears to be a lifelong challenge in which the individual must vigilantly "be aware and be active" in terms of identifying, modifying, and interacting with the listening environment. Therapy has not provided a magic pill or permanent solution to the symptoms. Depending on the diagnosis and other contributing factors, therapy in its formal sense may be relatively short in duration, while in other cases therapy may be more protracted or perhaps supportive in nature. In any event, therapy can be viewed as the device by which the students are placed on the right path. However, the path may be quite long and tortuous, and students must provide their own transportation. Without personal, ongoing responsibility and effort, the positive effects experienced in formal therapy may be shortlived; but with responsibility and effort, these students often can carry on "normal" lives.

In many cases the speech-language pathologist is available for consultations after discharge from therapy. Students may use the speech-language pathologist as a means of overseeing skill maintenance or as a source of information when questions or concerns arise. However, since the ultimate goal in therapy is independence, eventually students should not need this resource. At that point, the students are their own resources, fully capable of employing whatever strategies are needed, in whatever setting, in order to succeed.

Attitude thus becomes the essential element in transition. The ongoing need for vigilance and participation may be viewed from a negative perspective or approached much the same as the need to wear glasses or other prostheses. ("Poor me. I have to wear these ugly glasses"; or "Glasses make my life much easier and I'm glad to have them. Before I got my glasses I didn't see very well and missed so much of what was going on around me. Wearing them is a small price for the benefits they give me.")

Help transitioning students to realize that all of us at some point in our lives must rely on a prothesis, a tool, a procedure, or some other means of aid. One can choose to deny the need for a support system and live with the negative effects, or look at the situation realistically and live more fully. It is a choice not unlike other life choices to be made, some of which impact very dramatically upon the quality of one's life.

Carryover of skills is always a major concern in any therapy. When therapists recognize the need for progression of skill applications to more and more challenging and naturalistic settings and tasks, many of these concerns are reduced. If the final focuses of therapy involve the use of skills and strategies in the classroom, in the cafeteria, on the playground, and on the telephone, then carryover is more assured. Therapy and carryover blend together. Therapy is not some remote process that takes place in a small room, but a dynamic, evolving process that may start off in a small room but end on the playground. Similarly, therapy may have begun on a one-to-one basis, child and therapist, and progressed to interactions with several therapy partners. When therapy is designed and constructed individually with a goal toward independent functioning, it is likely to incorporate carryover within the long-range plan itself.

This is accomplished easily when therapy is seen in terms of "the big picture" or "What does this child need right now in order to ultimately be able to function without therapy? What skills, strategies, and attitudes can I build now that will allow this child to succeed as an adult?" Ask these questions daily. Perhaps our interests and responsibilities as therapists should exceed the prescriptions of the IEP or other legal mandates in the sense of goals. When accountability for relatively short-term focuses becomes paramount and exclusive, it is sometimes easy to lose focus of what the real point is in therapy.

The following list of suggestions for transitioning may be helpful for both the child with CAPD and the child's parents.

Transition from Therapy to Independence

1. The child must learn to modify his or her own listening environment (using preferential seating, looking at the speaker's face, and so on).

2. The child must be aware that *listening* (different from *hearing*) is an active process that requires responsibility and effort.

3. The child must be aware that skills learned in therapy must be continuously activated and applied. Once learned does not mean present permanently.

4. Continual monitoring of skills is vital. Rescreening of skills may be needed.

5. If skills have not been maintained, occasional brief periods of therapy may be needed.

6. Parents and teachers may use therapy folder materials as a basis for reinforcement. New materials may be added as recommended by the speech-language pathologist.

7. Parents and teachers should continue to use strategies (expressive tone of voice, auditory mirroring, reducing background noise, rephrasing, and others).

8. The child must continuously apply strategies (subvocalization, reauditorization, and others).

9. The status of hearing acuity may need to be frequently monitored by the audiologist.

10. The status of academic subjects—especially reading, spelling, and foreign languages—must be monitored. These areas are particularly sensitive to auditory processing skill status.

11. Since focus is on the "whole child" and not simply auditory processing skill development, psychological, physical, and social concerns must be addressed. Maintenance of health in all areas is important.

12. Continual contact with all concerned participants (classroom teacher, audiologist, physician, speech-language pathologist), even after the point of discharge from therapy, is recommended. However, eventually independent functioning is desirable.

Letter to Parents or Guardians

The following is a sample letter designed to inform parents about central auditory processing therapy.

- -

Date: _____

Dear _____:

Since our recent Committee of Special Education meeting, you may have some questions about central auditory processing therapy.

In children who have central auditory processing disorders (CAPD), the ears may function well, but the central nervous system may not effectively process what is heard. Therapy helps these children learn better ways to use what they hear.

As many as 14 skills are involved in processing what is heard. Think of these skills as foundation tools for success in the classroom. For example, we may work to improve *auditory figure-ground skills*—the ability to screen out classroom noises and focus on the teacher's voice. Another skill is *auditory memory*—the ability to recall numbers, words, directions, and other information. This skill helps the child to remember lecture materials and follow directions.

Your child will learn to use some coping techniques and make some simple changes in the listening environment. Gradually your child will learn to take more and more responsibility for modifying and controlling the listening environment. The child becomes an active participant.

Your child's therapy goals are stated in the Individualized Education Program (the IEP). We will be discussing these goals in detail next time we meet.

We are eager to have you participate in your child's program. You are an important member of the team. Within the next few weeks, I will send you information about techniques and strategies you can use at home to help your child.

Please contact me at any time if you have any comments or questions. I will call you about our next meeting soon. I am looking forward to a very productive school year.

Thank you.

Sincerely,

_____

Speech-Language Pathologist

Central Auditory Processing Disorder / Dorothy A. Kelly, D.A. / ISBN 0761631623

Letter to Physician

- -

Date: _____

Dear Dr. _____:

_____ receives speech-language services for
    (child's name)
central auditory processing disorder at _____
              (school)

in _____.
    (town)

As a speech-language pathologist working with this child, I would like to share some recent assessment findings. The child's parent, _____, has given permission for this disclosure.

This child exhibits central auditory processing disorders in the following areas:

_____

_____

_____

These disorders may have negatively impacted on the child's classroom performance, particularly in the areas of:

_____

_____

_____

Hearing, allergies, and other health issues are of great concern in our program. I am very interested in any input you are able to share. Please contact me at _____ if you have any comments or questions.

Thank you for your interest.

Sincerely,

_____

Speech-Language Pathologist

Central Auditory Processing Disorder / Dorothy A. Kelly, D.A. / ISBN 0761631623

Letter to Audiologist

Date: _____

Dear _____ :

As you may know, _____ is being seen for central auditory
(child's name)

processing disorder at _____ in _____ .
(school)   (town)

I am a speech-language pathologist working with this child. I would like to share
some recent assessment findings. The child's parent, _____ ,
has given permission for this disclosure.

This child exhibits central auditory processing disorders in the following areas:

_____

_____

_____

This diagnosis was completed through use of the following assessment
procedures:

_____

_____

_____

These disorders have negatively impacted upon classroom performance, particularly in the areas of:

_____

_____

Hearing and middle-ear status are of great concern in our program. I am very
interested in any input you are able to share. Please contact me at _____
if you have any comments or questions.

Thank you for your cooperation.

Sincerely,

_____
Speech-Language Pathologist

A Look to the Future

Although we are beginning to understand central auditory processing disorders in their many forms, much is left to learn. The following list identifies some areas of concern for future research and clinical focus.

1. Establish better means of identifying at-risk infants and children.

2. Establish more norm-referenced screening procedures.

3. Develop better assessment procedures for adolescents and adults.

4. Develop better assessment procedures for very young children.

5. Develop more therapy materials and strategies for children, adolescents, and adults.

6. Further investigate the effects of hearing loss (transitory or permanent) on central auditory processing.

7. Learn more about central auditory processing disorders in adolescence and adulthood.

8. Further investigate the relationship between central auditory processing and language development.

9. Further investigate the relationship between central auditory processing development and factors such as environment, sex, and maturation.

10. Learn more about the relationships between central auditory processing disorders and attention deficit disorder, learning disabilities, and similar conditions.

11. Further clarify the relationship between chronic otitis media and central auditory processing disorders.

12. Provide more information and a broader range of clinical experiences on the master's degree level in terms of central auditory processing disorders.

13. Discover more effective means of coordinating information and efforts with other professionals (physician, classroom teacher, psychologist, and others).

14. Further investigate etiological factors for the purposes of intervention and prevention.

15. Explore the possibility of processing delays versus disorders in terms of both etiology and intervention issues.

Discharge from Therapy

Name:

Date:

Grade/Placement:

Classroom Teacher:

Speech-Language Pathologist:

Status of Central Auditory Processing Skills:

_____

_____

_____

_____

_____

_____

_____

Reason(s) for Discharge:

_____

_____

_____

_____

_____

_____

_____

Recommendations/Follow-up:

_____

_____

_____

_____

_____

_____

_____

_____

_____
Speech-Language Pathologist

Appendix, Glossary, References

Checklist of Auditory Perceptual Subskills

The following checklist may be helpful in assessing very young children or older, significantly involved populations. View the items as foundation behaviors that suggest more mature auditory perceptual skills to follow.

Just as the auditory perceptual skill areas described in this book may be thought of as foundation tools for language development, the behaviors listed in the checklist are foundation tools for auditory perceptual skill area development. The behaviors noted have cognitive, social, and linguistic underpinnings. The checklist may be used as part of a diagnostic evaluation with infants and toddlers as well as with significantly delayed populations (for example, those with pervasive developmental delay).

Checklist of Auditory Perceptual Subskills

Name:	Date:

Key:
CO = Consistently observable
NO = Not observed
IO = Questionable or inconsistently observed

	CO	NO	IO
1. Appears to recognize familiar sounds.			
2. Appears to recognize familiar voices.			
3. Responds differentially to voices (for example, may be quieted by parent's voice).			
4. Responds grossly to intonation cues in voices.			
5. Attempts to imitate sounds heard.			
6. Exhibits intonation variation in own vocalizations.			
7. Appears to associate sounds with sound sources (for example, barking/dog).			
8. Seeks to localize sound sources.			
9. Appears to enjoy particular sounds (for example, bells, music).			
10. Displays a variety of vocalized sounds.			
11. Can maintain auditory attention for at least 30 seconds.			
12. Attends to people when speaking.			
13. Vocalizes when playing.			
14. Appears to anticipate sounds associated with favored activities (for example, eating, going out in car, watching television).			
15. Can be quieted by favored sounds (for example, singing, music).			
16. Responds to name.			
17. Reacts appropriately to sudden loud noises.			
18. Appears to react differentially to noises (for example, soft music versus loud cafeteria noises).			
19. Appears to attend to auditory stimuli differentially (maintaining longer attention to preferred sounds).			
20. Has demonstrated increasing subskills as noted above.			

Comments:

Central Auditory Processing Disorder / Dorothy A. Kelly, D.A. / ISBN 0761631623

Glossary

Assistive listening device—Any instrumentation that improves auditory functioning (hearing aids, 3-D Loop Assistive Listening System, and so on). May be part of a comprehensive aural rehabilitation program.

Auditory attention—The ability to maintain focus over a period of time for an intended purpose. Issues of neurology, volitionality, and interest become relevant. Appears related in part to other skills such as auditory memory and other factors such as maturation and interest.

Auditory cohesion—The ability to interpret, organize, and synthesize auditory information on a higher-order level of functioning. May be related to other skills such as auditory memory. Related to terms such as integration and organization (Katz 1989), synthesis, critical listening, categorization, and others.

Auditory discrimination—The ability to identify or note phonemic differences between sounds or words. Related to tasks such as following directions, spelling, reading decoding, and writing.

Auditory figure-ground—The ability to identify or focus on the primary auditory signal in the presence of secondary or background signals. Relates to classroom functioning and the ability to carry out directions and maintain focus. Also known as auditory separation and auditory selective attention.

Auditory integration training—Treatment programs which use auditory stimulation techniques to reduce hypersensitivity and improve listening skills in patients with complex communication, learning, and behavior difficulties.

Auditory latency—A lapse or delay in response time when presented with auditory input.

Auditory memory—The ability to recall numbers of units (words, numbers, sentences, phonemes, and so on). Related to auditory sequential memory (recall of units in a particular sequence) as well as the ability to interpret directions (which involves accurate memory as well as appropriate response or action). Can be assessed in terms of immediate and deferred recall and response.

Auditory mirroring—Technique wherein therapist, teacher, or parent can provide reinforcement, modeling, and/or clarification to the child with CAPD by returning utterances produced by the child in appropriate form and/or expanded form.

Auditory perception—A term described in a variety of ways but generally related to sound/symbol associations and the comprehension of sounds and words; the endpoint of auditory processing (Sloan 1991). Appears related to auditory discrimination.

Auditory trainers—Instruments to improve auditory functioning; used by persons with hearing impairment or auditory perceptual impairment. Designed for a variety of purposes (including auditory figure-ground difficulties) depending on the population and setting involved.

Auditory-visual integration—The simultaneous processing of sound and sight. Often involves symbolic functions.

Central auditory nervous system—The pathway that an auditory signal takes enroute to the brain once it has exited the ear (peripheral hearing system).

Central auditory processing—Interpretation and manipulation of verbal and nonverbal auditory signals on a meaningful basis beyond the peripheral hearing system (ear level).

Central auditory processing disorders—A variety of impairments, primary or secondary in nature, that involve an inability to respond to auditory stimuli effectively. Not due to impairments of hearing sensitivity or intellect. Based beyond the peripheral ear system.

Chunking—A memory strategy in which the child is encouraged to recall specific words through associations or clusters of related words. Modified here to involve volume and intonation cues (see page 140).

Otitis media—An infection of the middle ear cavity often involving conductive hearing loss. Frequently recurrent; a common childhood condition.

Peripheral hearing—Auditory sensitivity that is measurable by audiometry and based within the ear itself.

Reauditorization—One of 14 auditory processing skills identified by Heasley (1974, 31) and described as higher-order recollection of sound on a thought level. As used here, a strategy employed to aid auditory memory and interpretation of directions, among other tasks.

Subvocalization—As used in this text, subvocalization is an adaptation of the procedure described by Heasley (1974, 30-31). Whereas Heasley advocated repetition without sound (mouthing), this text recommends repetition with vocalization to reinforce auditory processing. It is a vocalized strategy used to aid auditory memory and the interpretation of directions, among other tasks. Considered to be similar to, but of a lower order than, reauditorization because it is completed on a vocalized level, whereas reauditorization involves thought processes only.

References

Abbs, J. H., and H. M. Sussman. 1971. Neurophysiological feature detectors and speech perception: A discussion of theoretical implications. *Journal of Speech and Hearing Research* 14:23-36.

Allen, D. V., and D. O. Robinson. 1984. Middle ear status and language development in preschool children. *Asha* June:33-37.

American Speech-Language-Hearing Association. 1992. *Issues in central auditory processing disorders: A report from the ASHA Ad Hoc Committee on Central Auditory Processing,* Gail Chermak, chair. Rockville, MD: American Speech-Language-Hearing Association.

Bankson, N. 1977. *Bankson language screening test* (manual). Baltimore: University Park Press.

Berard, G. 1993. *Hearing equals behaving.* New Canaan, CT: Keats.

Berko-Gleason, J. 1983. Otitis media and language development. *Pediatrics* 71:644-45.

Berry, M. F. 1960. *Language development of children.* New York: Appleton- Century- Crofts.

Boone, D. R. 1987. *Human communication and its disorders.* Englewood Cliffs, NJ: Prentice Hall.

Borrild, K. 1978. Classroom acoustics. In *Auditory management of hearing impaired children,* edited by M. Ross and T. Giolas, 147-79. Baltimore: University Park Press.

Delgutte, B. 1980. Representation of speech-like sounds in the discharge patterns of auditory nerve fibers. *Journal of the Acoustical Society of America* 63:843-57.

Dunn, L., and L. M. Dunn. 1981. *Peabody picture vocabulary test—Revised.* Circle Pines, MN: American Guidance Service.

Eisenson, J. 1966. Perceptual disturbances in children with central nervous system disfunctions and implications for language development. *British Journal of Disorders in Communication* 1(1): 21-32.

_____. 1972. *Aphasia in children.* London: Harper and Row.

Friel-Patti, S. 1990. Otitis media with effusion and the development of language: A review of the evidence. *Topics in Language Disorders* 2(1):11-22.

Friel-Patti, S., and T. Finitzo. 1990. Language learning in a prospective study of otitis media with effusion in the first two years of life. *Journal of Speech and Hearing Research* 33(1):188-94.

Gardner, M. F. 1979. *Expressive one-word picture vocabulary test.* Novato, CA: Academic Therapy Publications.

_____. 1983. *Expressive one-word picture vocabulary test (upper extension).* Novato, CA: Academic Therapy Publications.

_____. 1985. *Test of auditory perceptual skills.* San Francisco: Children's Hospital of San Francisco.

_____. 1993. *Test of auditory reasoning and processing skills.* Burlingame, CA: Psychological and Educational Publications.

Garrand, K. R., and B. S. Clark. 1985. Otitis media: The role of speech-language pathologists. *Asha* 27(7):35-40.

Gillet, P. 1993. *Auditory processes—Revised ed.* Novato, CA: Academic Therapy Publications.

Giolas, T. G. 1986. *Aural rehabilitation.* Austin, TX: Pro-Ed.

Goldman, R., M. Fristoe, and R. W. Woodcock. 1970. *Test of auditory discrimination.* Circle Pines, MN: American Guidance Service.

Gottlieb, M., and P.W. Zinkus. 1980. Patterns of perceptual and academic deficits related to early chronic otitis media. *Pediatrics* 64:246-252

Gravel, J. S., and I. F. Wallace. 1992. Listening and language at 4 years of age: Effects of early otitis media. *Journal of Speech and Hearing Research* 35(3): 588-95.

Grievink, E. H., S. A. F. Peters, W. H. J. van Bon, and A. G. M. Schilder. 1993. The effects of early bilateral otitis media with effusion on language ability: A prospective cohort study. *Journal of Speech and Hearing Research* 36(5): 1004-12.

Hart, P. J. 1983. Classroom acoustical environments for children with central auditory processing disorders. In *Central auditory processing disorders— Problems of speech, language and learning,* edited by E. Lasky and J. Katz, 343-52. Baltimore: University Park Press.

Heasley, B. E. 1974. *Auditory perceptual disorders and remediation.* Springfield, IL: Charles C. Thomas.

Howie, V. M., J. H. Ploussard, and J. Sloyer. 1975. The "otitis prone" condition. *American Journal of Diseases in Children* 129:676-78.

Jerger, J., and S. Jerger. 1971. Diagnostic significance of PB word functions. *Archives of Otolaryngology* 93(197):573-80.

Jerger, S., J. Jerger, B.R. Alford, and S. Abrams. 1983. Development of speech intelligibility in children with recurrent otitis media. *Ear and Hearing* 4:138-145.

Katz, J. 1968. The SSW test: An interim report. *Journal of Speech and Hearing Disorders* 33:132-46.

_____. 1977. The staggered spondaic word test. In *Central auditory dysfunction,* edited by R. Keith. New York: Grune and Stratton.

_____. 1989. *Diagnostic report.* Personal communication.

Kelly, D. 1993a. Otitis media: An increasingly prevalent and confusing phenomenon. *Advance for Speech-Language Pathologists and Audiologists* 3(2):9.

_____. 1993b. Dyslexia and the inner ear: Innovative treatment combines therapy and medication. *Advance for Speech-Language Pathologists and Audiologists* 3(24):10-11.

Kiang, N. Y. S. 1980. Processing of speech by the auditory nervous system. *Journal of the Acoustical Society of America* 63:830-35.

Klein, J. O. 1983. Epidemiology and natural history of otitis media. *Pediatrics* 71:639-40.

Lasky, E. Z., and J. Katz. 1983. Perspectives on central auditory processing. In *Central auditory processing disorders—Problems of speech, language and learning*, edited by E. Z. Lasky and J. Katz, 3-10. Baltimore: University Park Press.

Lenneberg, E. H. 1967. *Biological foundations of language*. New York: John Wiley.

Leslie, L., and J. Caldwell. 1990. *Qualitative reading inventory*. London: Scott, Foresman.

Leverett, R. G., and A. D. Diefendorf. 1992. Students with language deficiencies—Suggestions for frustrated teachers. *Teaching Exceptional Children* 24:30-35.

Lindamood, C. H., and P. C. Lindamood. 1975. *Auditory discrimination in depth program*, rev. ed. Boston: Teaching Resources.

Lubert, N. 1981. Auditory perceptual impairment in children with specific language disorders: A review of the literature. *Journal of Speech and Hearing Disorders* 46:3-9.

Martin, F. N. 1986. *Introduction to audiology*. Englewood Cliffs, NJ: Prentice Hall.

Matkin, N. D., and P. E. Hook. 1983. A multidisciplinary approach to central auditory evaluations. In *Central auditory processing disorders—Problems of speech, language and learning*, edited by E. Z. Lasky and J. Katz, 223-42. Baltimore: University Park Press.

Menyuk, P. 1980. Effects of persistent otitis media on language development. *Annals of Otology, Rhinology and Laryngology* 89(3):257-63.

Musiek, F. E., N. A. Guerkink, and S. A. Keitel. 1982. Test battery assessment of auditory perceptual dysfunction in children. *Laryngoscope* 92:251-57.

Musiek, F. E., S. Lenz, and K. M. Gollegly. 1991. Neuroaudiology correlates to anatomical changes of the brain. *American Journal of Audiology* 1:19-24.

Neuman, A. C., and I. Hochberg. 1983. Children's perception of speech in reverberation. *Journal of the Acoustical Society of America* 73:2145-49.

Newby, H. A. 1972. *Audiology*, 3d ed. New York: Appleton-Century-Crofts.

Newcomer, Phyllis L., and Donald D. Hammill. 1982. *Test of language development—Primary*. Austin, TX: Pro-Ed.

Northern, J. L., and M. L. Lemme. 1988. Hearing and auditory disorders. In *Human communication disorders*, 2nd ed., edited by G. Shames and E. Wiig, 415-44. Columbus, OH: Charles E. Merrill.

O'Brien, D. 1993. Issues in aural rehabilitation. *Lex Talk Newsletter* 1:1.

Paradise, J. L. 1980. Otitis media in infants and children. *Pediatrics* 65:917-43.

Paul, R., T. F. Lynn, and M. Lohr-Flanders. 1993. History of middle ear involvement and speech/language development in late talkers. *Journal of Speech and Hearing Research* 36:1055-62.

Physician survey: Parents need to be educated about pediatric ear infections. 1994. *Advance for Speech-Language Pathologists and Audiologists* 4(25) October 24:8.

Pinheiro, M. L. 1977. Tests of central auditory function in children with learning disabilities. In *Central auditory dysfunction,* edited by R. Keith, 223-56. New York: Grune and Stratton.

Pinheiro, M. L., and F. E. Musiek. 1985a. Dichotic speech tests in detection of central auditory dysfunction. In *Assessment of central auditory dysfunctions: Foundations and clinical correlates,* edited by M. L. Pinheiro and F. E. Musiek, 201-17. Baltimore: Williams and Wilkins.

_____. 1985b. Special considerations in central auditory evaluation. In *Assessment of central auditory dysfunctions: Foundations and clinical correlates,* edited by M. L. Pinheiro and F. E. Musiek, 257-65. Baltimore: Williams and Wilkins.

Quick, C., and C. Mandell. 1983. *Otitis media and learning disabilities: More than a relationship?* Paper presented at the 61st Annual International Convention of the Council for Exceptional Children, Detroit.

Reichman, J., and W. C. Healey. 1983. Learning disabilities and conductive hearing loss involving otitis media. *Journal of Learning Disabilities* 16(5): 272-78.

Rimland, B. 1992. *Autism Research Institute Newsletter.* San Diego: CA: Autism Research Institute.

Roberts, J. E., M. R. Burchinal, M. A. Koch, M. M. Footo, and F. W. Henderson. 1988. Otitis media in early childhood and its relationship to later phonological development. *Journal of Speech and Hearing Disorders* 53(4): 424-32.

Roberts, J. E., M. R. Burchinal, B. P. Davis, A. M. Collier, and F. W. Henderson. 1991. Otitis media in early childhood and later language. *Journal of Speech and Hearing Research* 34:1158-68.

Rosenthal, W. S. 1977. The role of perception in child language disorders. *Communicative Disorders: An Audio Journal for Continuing Education* 2(7) (audiocassette). New York: Grune and Stratton.

Ross, M. 1978. Classroom acoustics and speech intelligibility. In *Handbook of clinical audiology,* edited by J. Katz, 469-78. Baltimore: Williams and Wilkins.

Scaldwell, William A. 1985. Prevalence of otitis media in Cree and Ojibway school children in six Ontario communities. *Journal of American Indian Education* 25(1) November:1-5.

Shurin, P. A., S. I. Pelton, A. Donner, and J. O. Klein. 1979. Persistence of middle ear effusion after acute otitis media in children. *New England Journal of Medicine* 300:1121-23.

Silvaroli, N. 1983. *Classroom reading inventory.* Dubuque, IA: William C. Brown.

Skinner, M. W. 1978. Electroencephalic response audiometry. In *Handbook of clinical audiology,* edited by J. Kavanagh, 311-24. Baltimore: Williams and Wilkins.

Sloan, C. 1980. Auditory processing disorders and language development. In *Auditory processing and language: Clinical and research perspectives,* edited by P. J. Levinson and C. Sloan, 101-16. New York: Grune and Stratton.

_____. 1991. *Treating auditory processing difficulties in children.* San Diego: Singleton.

Stehli, A. 1991. *The sound of a miracle: A child's triumph over autism.* New York: Doubleday.

Sudler, W. H., and C. Flexer. 1986. Low cost assistive listening device. *Language, Speech and Hearing Services in Schools* 17(4):342-44.

Tallal, P. 1980. Auditory processing disorders in children. In *Auditory processes and language: Clinical and research perspectives,* edited by P. J. Levinson and C. Sloan, 81-100. New York: Grune and Stratton.

Tallal, P., and R. E. Stark. 1981. Speech acoustic-cue discrimination abilities of normally developing and language-impaired children. *Journal of the Acoustical Society of America* 69:568-74.

Tallal, P., R. E. Stark, C. Kallman, and D. Mellitis. 1980. Developmental dysphasia: Relationship between acoustic processing and verbal processing. *Neuropsychologia* 18:273-84.

Terman, L., and M. Merrill. 1960. *Stanford-Binet intelligence scale.* Boston: Houghton-Mifflin.

Trace R. 1993a. CAPD diagnosis requires comprehensive assessment. *Advance for Speech-Language Pathologists and Audiologists* 3(16):7, 13.

_____. 1993b. Researchers, clinicians discuss a "healthy" diversity of approaches to CAPD. *Advance for Speech-Language Pathologists and Audiologists* 3(16):10, 11, 13.

Ventry, I. M. 1980. Effects of conductive hearing loss: Fact or fiction? *Journal of Speech and Hearing Disorders* 45:143-56.

Willeford, J. 1977. Assessing central auditory behavior in children: A test battery approach. In *Central auditory dysfunction,* edited by R. Keith, 1-42. New York: Grune and Stratton.

_____. 1985. Assessment of central auditory disorders in children. In *Assessment of central auditory dysfunctions—foundations and clinical correlates,* edited by M. L. Pinheiro and F. E. Musiek, 239-55. Baltimore: Williams and Wilkins.

Wyngaarden, J. B., Chairman, Interaging Committee on Learning Disabilities. 1987. *Learning disabilities—A report to the U.S. Congress* 168. Washington, DC: Government Printing Office.

Zinkus, P. 1986. Perceptual and academic deficits related to early chronic otitis media. In *Otitis media and child development,* edited by J. Kavanagh, 107-16. Parkton, MD: York.